Gilles Paquet and Roger A. Perrault

The Tainted-Blood Tragedy in Canada

A Cascade of Governance Failures

Collaborative Decentred Metagovernance Series

This series of books is designed to define cumulatively the contours of collaborative decentred metagovernance. At this time, there is still no canonical version of this paradigm: it is *en émergence*. This series intends to be one of many 'construction sites' to experiment with various dimensions of an effective and practical version of this new approach.

Metagovernance is the art of combining different forms or styles of governance, experimented with in the private, public and social sectors, to ensure effective coordination when power, resources and information are widely distributed, and the governing is of necessity decentred and collaborative.

The series invites conceptual and practical contributions focused on different issue domains, policy fields, *causes célèbres*, functional processes, etc. to the extent that they contribute to sharpening the new apparatus associated with collaborative decentred metagovernance.

In the last few decades, there has been a need felt for a more sophisticated understanding of the governing of the private, public and social sectors: for less compartmentalization among sectors that have much in common; and for new conceptual tools to suggest new relevant questions and new ways to carry out the business of governing, by creatively recombining the tools of governance that have proven successful in all these sectors. These efforts have generated experiments that have been sufficiently rich and wide-ranging in the various laboratories to warrant efforts to pull together what we know at this stage.

This tenth volume in the series revisits the tainted-blood tragedy that Canada experienced in the latter part of the 20th century. It presents an argument in brief about the tragedy being the result of a cascade of pathologies of governance. Then it challenges the conventional wisdom and its explanation, boiling it down to four ill-founded accusations. After proposing a systemic reconstruction of the tragedy, it develops some responses to the systemic governance failures. The conclusion takes stock of the modest progress in the repairs of the toxic system in place, and the postface focuses on both the demise of critical thinking as a fundamental source of the crisis and on a need to refurbish critical thinking if advances are to be expected in what remains a work in progress.

Interested parties are invited to join the Chautauqua.

– Editorial Board

Other titles published by INVENIRE are listed at the end of the book.

Gilles Paquet and Roger A. Perrault

The Tainted-Blood Tragedy in Canada

A Cascade of Governance Failures

INVENIRE

Ottawa, Canada
2016

Invenire © 2016

Library and Archives Canada Cataloguing in Publication

Paquet, Gilles, 1936-, author
    The tainted-blood tragedy in Canada : a cascade of
governance failures / by Gilles Paquet and Roger A. Perrault.

Issued in print and electronic formats.
ISBN 978-1-927465-30-1 (paperback).--ISBN 978-1-927465-31-8
(html)

        1. Blood banks--Canada--Quality control. 2. Blood banks--
Risk management--Canada. I. Perrault, Roger A., 1936-, author
II. Title.

RM172.P34 2016   362.17'840971   C2016-901142-9
                                               C2016-901143-7

Invenire would like to gratefully acknowledge the ongoing support for this
series by the Centre on Governance, University of Ottawa.

Published by Invenire
P.O. Box 87001
Ottawa, Canada K2P 1X0
www.invenire.ca

Cover design by Sandy Lynch
Layout and design by Sandy Lynch
Printed in Canada by Imprimerie Gauvin

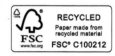

RECYCLED
Paper made from
recycled material
FSC
www.fsc.org   FSC® C100212

Distributed by:
Commoners' Publishing
631 Tubman Cr.
Ottawa, Canada K1V 8L6
Tel.: 613-523-2444
Fax: 888-613-0329
sales@commonerspublishing.com
www.commonerspublishing.com

| Table of Contents

Tu n'as rien vu à Hiroshima
Marguerite Duras

PREFACE

This short book has been written by a specialist on governance, and a medical doctor and scientist who managed the Canadian blood transfusion system for 17 years (1974-91). It is about a tragedy that has left a number of Canadians dead, and a larger number incapacitated or seriously handicapped.

One of us (Dr. Roger A. Perrault), former National Director of the Canadian Red Cross, Blood Transfusion Service, has been accused of having been at fault, and having to shoulder some responsibility for this tragedy because of delays in appropriate action being taken. It is a matter that, following a lengthy RCMP investigation, led to criminal charges that have now been examined by the courts. Dr. Perrault has been fully exonerated on all counts. Indeed, Justice Mary Lou Benotto of the Superior Court of Ontario stated this clearly in her judgment acquitting Dr. Perrault on October 1st, 2007:

> Far from establishing the requirements of either negligence or nuisance, the Crown has persuaded me that Dr. Perrault acted carefully and reasonably in regard to the health and safety of hemophiliacs in Canada. He worked diligently in the interest of the hemophiliac community.
>
> He hired leading experts to work with him at the National Office and in the regional centres. He relied on the regulatory authorities and was in consultation with them on all the important decisions. They were forced to choose between distributing a product that was not risk free and leaving hemophiliacs without a life-saving treatment. He was put in a position of immense public trust.

In that capacity he was thrust into a series of difficult events to which he responded with care, thoughtfulness and utmost professionalism (see Part II of this volume).

So this book is not about vindicating the character and behaviour of Dr. Perrault. That has already been done very decisively by the court.

Yet, even if it has been established that there was no criminal negligence or nuisance, there were most certainly governance failures, and this latter aspect of the tragedy has neither received the attention it deserves, nor has the limited attention it received led to much social learning or to suggestions about governance repairs that might mitigate the damages the next time the unthinkable strikes.

There has been much hand-wringing and irresponsible rhetoric over the years about the tainted-blood affair, and much scapegoating, but little written about what should be learned from the whole affair:

- about governance in the face of deep uncertainty;
- about flaws in Canadian governance institutions, and the breakdown of collaborative interprovincial governance that was witnessed;
- about the failures of the processes that were unleashed in the wake of the blood tragedy; and
- about certain features of the Canadian psyche that were revealed when the media, the public and the authorities attempted to come to grips with the tainted-blood tragedy.

The sort of reconstruction of events that this book has undertaken of what occurred over 25 years is of necessity fraught with possibilities of information being difficult to secure, of key witnesses having passed away, of documentation being difficult to secure, and of difficulty in reconciling the different incompatible interpretations of agonistic events. This has called for particular care in establishing the basic facts of the case, in critically appraising the conventional wisdom that has come to be somewhat irresponsibly accepted as truth by the media, and in developing a line of argument damning governance in our explanation of a more satisfactory account of this tragedy.

Over and beyond the persons and groups that are mentioned explicitly in the body of the text, certain individuals were of considerable help in providing information or confirmation about a variety of aspects of our argument. We would like to express our gratitude to the large number of persons who, in different ways, have been helpful during the long period of gestation of this book. A few individuals deserve to be identified by name for their help, but this is done while at the same time exculpating them in advance for whatever use we have made of their contribution.

From the Canadian Red Cross Blood Transfusion Service:

Dr. Morris Blajchman, former Medical Director of the Hamilton Blood Centre

Dr. James Strong, former Medical Director of the Sudbury Blood Centre

Mr. Stephen Vick, former Director, Blood Products Services

From the Canadian Blood Committee:

Ms. Elaine Boily, former member of the Canadian Blood Committee Secretariat

We are grateful for the latitude provided by the State in the reproduction of legal documents, while accepting that the copyright remains with the Superior of Justice. The copy of the judgment was provided by the office of Greenspan Partners (RAP's lawyers) following the 2006-07 trial when the judgment was handed down by Justice Benotto on October 1, 2007. The material in Part II of this book is an accurate version of the judgment, and is not to be used for commercial purposes.

Finally, a special word of thanks must be recorded for Mrs. Janet Perrault, the wife of Dr. Perrault, who was supportive not only during the period of production of this book, but also over the span of some 30 years during which the tainted-blood tragedy impacted her family.

As usual, McEvoy Galbreath and her team at Invenire must be complimented for making the last stages in the production of this book as effective and pleasant as possible. The editorial assistance of Anne Burgess is also much appreciated.

PART I

INTRODUCTION

| *Factum, Explanandum* and *Explanans*

This book intends to provide a compendium of three sets of information. First, it wishes to communicate to a broad public a set of information about the tainted-blood tragedy in Canada: what lawyers call the *factum* – an ensemble of facts that are not disputed by any party and constitute the basis on which the case rests; second, what we call the *explanandum* – what is to be explained – an ensemble of questions that would appear to remain unanswered or unsatisfactorily answered about the case; and third, what we call *explanans* – an explanation that we regard as more satisfactory.

In this introduction, we set the stage for our discussion by drawing attention to some key features and concerns that have been forgotten in handling wicked policy problems in a complex, turbulent and chaotic world like ours – where crises and avalanches are to be expected.

The notion of wicked problems has been suggested by Rittel and Webber (1973) and has been defined by Valerie Brown and colleagues (Brown *et al.* 2010: 4) as follows:

A wicked problem is a complex issue that defies complete definition, for which there can be no final solution, since any resolution generates further issues, and where solutions are not true or false or good or bad but the best that can be done at the time. Such problems are not morally wicked, but diabolical in that they resist all the usual attempts to resolve them.

Such problems require a new approach to the conduct of research, and call for different forms of governance and changes in ways of living. This, in turn, requires a more open, transdisciplinary and exploratory sort of inquiry.

Collective actions cannot be legitimized solely by the evocation of the good intentions of those involved. Risk acceptability is often more dependent upon the dogmas of distributive justice than upon the perception of risk magnitude (Renn 2008: xiv). One of the most resilient of these dogmas is the stubborn and unreasonable belief that 100 percent safety can and should be guaranteed in our evolving complex and turbulent world, even though it is eminently clear that it cannot be guaranteed even in the best of circumstances. The quest for zero-risk is laudable, but utopian: it is a futile and illusory quest. The best one can hope for is transparency and professionalism in coping with ever more daunting challenges, in ensuring that social learning proceeds as fast as possible, and that lessons learned reduce the magnitude of harms in the future.

On the governance front

It has become clear that human contraptions (organizations and institutions) are fallible. They are usually fragmented (as power, resources and information are widely distributed), depend on expert opinions and lay perceptions, and are always torn by often contradictory ethical and technical imperatives. In the social arena of governance in the face of uncertainty, everything happens in real time, and therefore trade-offs are constantly redefined among different perceptions and threats. What is at stake, and therefore evaluable, is the 'collective judgment' and 'trustworthiness' of the system.

Both the blood transfusion system and the media-lobbies-political (MLP) system have given signs of governance failures. In the first place, the structure in place was flawed, and it led to dysfunctions – a public health enterprise based on presumptive collaborative governance was marred by disunity and inter-agency tensions that prevented the blood transfusion system from operating as well as it might have. In the second place, the

MLP processes revealed an immense sensitivity to disruptive forces: victims' lobbying influencing uncritical media, bringing much pressure on the political realm, and, as an echo effect, derailing the police investigation (no longer focused on fact finding, but rather on indicting) and the work of the Crown (to the point of preventing the Crown attorney from exercising sound judgment as to the evidence available). Much of the MLP system seemed to be determined to find guilty parties, and to seek punishment. For these *magistrats de l'immédiat* (instant indictors), but also for the police force and the Office of the Attorney General – all subjected to the immense pressure of victims and public opinion – the notion of 'systemic failure' appeared to be nothing but a sort of cop-out: personalized responsibility was demanded for all mishaps (McDuff 1995: 254). As a result, there was a temptation to ascribe the responsibility for the perceived governance failure of the Blood Transfusion Service to a person or persons who were seen as officials of the system.

On the inquiry and adjudicatory processes set up to determine evidence of negligence

These are most imperfect instruments. They most often prevent a full and meaningful review of the complex processes they are meant to probe, and they may too easily be hijacked by aggrieved parties, or distorted out of shape by the sensationalist and irresponsible ways of the media (Livermore 2010).

On the psyche front

The tainted-blood tragedy has illustrated two new features of our governance system: (1) the obsession with pinpointing blame and apportioning punishment when things go wrong, even when nobody is in charge, and when pinpointing responsibility may not only be difficult, but outright misguided; and (2) the tendency of governments to delegate the probing of such mishaps to all sorts of pseudo-expert bodies, operating under very loose rules of evidence, with the responsibility of adjudicating (quickly and on the basis of both a limited mandate and a snapshot approach to an evolving process) in cases of such complex and contentious issues. It is hardly surprising that such processes most often prove deeply flawed, even though the citizenry is prone to unwarrantedly grant much undeserved moral authority to the quasi-judicial personnel running such processes.

These features would appear to be in good currency in Canada, and to constitute major flaws that have often derailed our governance and our capacity for social learning (Paquet 2006; Hubbard and Paquet 2007).

It is our view that governance failures both upstream and downstream in the collective decision process need to be well understood and effectively corrected when they give signs of dysfunction. Indeed, it should be a constant priority. However, when crises entail human pain and death, much of the reaction to such tragedies is completely dominated by denunciations and emotion, fanned by the media and lobby groups. As a result, more attention is given to chronicling pain and apportioning blame than to diagnosing the governance failures and their sources, and correcting them. This is an unfortunate and toxic bias.

Continued improvement in an imperfect system

The intent of this book is not to deny, occlude or minimize the personal tragedy suffered by a large number of Canadians. Rather, its purpose is threefold.

First, it is to describe and explain the nature of the predicament faced by those charged with the management of the Blood Transfusion Service in the face of new emerging and not well-understood circumstances, as was the case on the occasion of the AIDS epidemic. Without a full appreciation of the complexity of the case and of the hyper-difficulty of the task, it is impossible for citizens to regain trust in the institutions that have served them well, although not with 100 percent certainty.

Second, it is to expound a cautionary tale about the way in which the tainted-blood tragedy was handled when it occurred, and about the fact that emotions came to trump due process, and to expose governance failures and also perspectives, ways and approaches that would appear to be toxic.

In a high-risk society that has become obsessed with accountability, but that lacks the full capacity to critically reflect on what it is doing (and therefore to self-correct when the governance system goes awry), governance failures of various sorts are likely to be numerous and costly. In particular, the obsessive search for a guilty party when there is a mishap has led the country to fall into the bad habits of using shoddy instruments like commissions of inquiry (set up with the noblest of intentions, but often degenerating into something akin to kangaroo courts and lynching parties) to adjudicate on these matters.

The accountability concerns, while understandable in the light of the horror of the human tragedies observed, fuel dangerous processes when commissions (like those conducted by Justice Krever or Justice Gomery, or others in the O'Connor and Iacobucci inquiries, to name some recent ones) unwarrantedly acquire a sort of moral authority and aura of infallibility they do not deserve. By their very nature, such inquiries "cannot afford as many safeguards as proceedings before a normal court of justice" (as Justice Gomery readily admitted in an interview with Jonathan Montpetit of *The Globe & Mail* on March 13, 2009).

As a result, these processes may also easily lead to incomplete appreciation and interpretation of facts, to erroneous conclusions (explicit or latent), and to scapegoating. The toxicity of the accountability obsession, and of the use of shoddy inquiry processes that thrive on 'mere plausibility' as their guiding norm, have bolstered the use of a new guidepost – **the precautionary principle**. This is a new dangerous, if popular, gauge to ascertain what the appropriate action is in complex circumstances.

To the extent that this new principle is simply a suggestion that prudence is *de rigueur*, this principle is innocuous, and indeed welcome. However, when it becomes 'judiciarized', and it purports to invent unreasonable standards – like the suggestion that persons should have been clairvoyant, that there is no limit to what officials should be expected to have anticipated, and that they should be held responsible for the tragedies generated not as a result of their not taking action on the basis of evidence, but on their not taking action as a matter of 'mandated clairvoyance' (Ewald *et al.* 2001; Paquet 2004: chapter 3) – the precautionary principle becomes toxic.

This new gospel is dangerous and challenges the very foundation of our democratic governance system: 'the presumption of innocence'. In the light of the use made of the precautionary principle by recently retired judges appointed to chair commissions of inquiry, commissions have come to be transmogrified into inquisitions; the burden of the proof has shifted onto the presumed innocent person to demonstrate that he or she had been sufficiently clairvoyant to meet this ill-defined, mandated level of warranted precaution. Perhaps more important, the use of such a gauge and the focus on blamableness have often derailed a process that should rather have focused mainly, if not single-mindedly, on the correction to the ever imperfect governance process.

Third, it is not sufficient to analyze the governance failures at the root of the tainted-blood tragedy. It is necessary to try to derive from these findings some suggestions on how to improve our governance systems to make them better able to cope with such occurrences of unpredictable and unthinkable public health crises (but also of like crises in other domains), for they are bound to recur (as the recent SARS and the H1N1 events have shown). We must therefore reflect on what has been learned about the tainted-blood tragedy, and the way in which it was handled *ex post*, that might be of use in ensuring that direct and collateral damages might be reduced next time (Ramo 2009).

These three general concerns have underpinned our work in this book.

The intent is not to deny that, with the benefit of hindsight, some might be seen as having shown poor judgment. Indeed, given what we know now, some things would clearly be done differently if faced with the same crisis. Our main concern, however, is to learn from the tainted-blood experience something that might help to improve the 'collective decision system' so as to make such tragedy less costly in human terms next time – both for the primary victims and for the secondary victims (i.e., those wrongfully and personally hounded for what were systemic governance failures).

In dealing with the tainted-blood tragedy, we proceed in four stages.

In chapter 1, we present our argument in brief about the tainted-blood tragedy being the result of a cascade of pathologies in governance. In chapter 2, we challenge the conventional wisdom that has proposed an explanation of the tragedy in terms of four ill-founded accusations. In chapter 3, we provide a systemic reconstruction and explanation of the tainted-blood tragedy in Canada. In chapter 4, we suggest a few modest general propositions that may be kept in mind in designing a response to systemic governance failures. Finally, in the conclusion, we take stock on the modest progress in the repairs of the toxic system in place. The postface underlines the demise of critical thinking as a profound cause of the little progress made in dealing with fundamental changes, and the importance of preserving loci where critical thinking is still highly regarded if advances are to be made in what remains a work in progress.

References

Brown, Valerie A. *et al.* (eds.). 2010. *Tackling Wicked Problems*. New York, NY: Earthscan.

Ewald, François, Christian Gollier and Nicolas de Sadeleer. 2001. *Le principe de précaution*. Paris, FR: Presses Universitaires de France.

Hubbard, Ruth and Gilles Paquet. 2007. *Gomery's Blinders and Canadian Federalism*. Ottawa, ON: The University of Ottawa Press.

Livermore, Daniel. 2010. "The Inquiry Model: Lessons from the O'Connor and Iacobucci Commissions," *www.optimumonline.ca*, 40(4): 1-28.

McDuff, Johanne. 1995. *Le sang qui tue.* Montreal, QC: Libre Expression.

Montpetit, Jonathan. 2009. "Gomery prepares to defend conclusions," *The Globe & Mail*, March 13.

O'Neill, Onora. 2002. *A Question of Trust.* Cambridge, UK: Cambridge University Press.

Paquet, Gilles. 2004. *Pathologies de gouvernance.* Montreal, QC: Liber.

Paquet, Gilles. 2006. "Une déprimante culture de l'adjudication," *Options Politiques*, 27(5): 40-45.

Ramo, Joshua C. 2009. *The Age of the Unthinkable.* New York, NY: Little Brown & Company.

Renn, Ortwin. 2008. *Risk Governance – Coping with Uncertainty in a Complex World.* London, UK: Earthscan.

Rittel, H. & M. Webber. 1973. "Dilemmas in a general theory of planning," *Policy Sciences*, 4: 155-169.

CHAPTER 1

A Cascade of Pathologies of Governance

On vous demande, quoi que vous fassiez, d'être en
mesure de prévenir un événement qui n'est pas prévisible,
mais dont on ne peut pas dire qu'il n'aura pas lieu.

Hubert Curien

T he basic objective of this chapter is to identify in a very stylized way the sort of 'mechanisms at work' in modern complex, socio-technical systems that might explain why errors occur, and how predictably irrational responses to such mishaps transform crises into tragedies, tragedies into scandals, and scandals into miscarriages of justice.

These mechanisms should in no way limit the ambit and scope of specific inquiries, which should not be restricted to the mechanical use of these effects, blockages and perspectives in the construction of an argument attempting to make sense of a tragedy. The template used should only serve as a provisional 'checklist' (Gawande 2009) to ensure that the existence of those too-often-ignored effects are not forgotten; one should neither feel the need to constantly refer to these mechanisms, nor to force empirical material through this issue-machine, as if they were compulsory figures.

This sequence of mechanisms is only one instrument to help deconstruct, in a provisional way, 'complex catastrophes as a cascade of pathologies'. The partial set of well-known mechanisms presented in the next section will serve as a helpful device to articulate how a cascade of mechanisms might work, and how one might articulate, elliptically, the study of complex catastrophes: a deconstruction of the tragedy as basically a cascade of governance mechanisms that failed.

Too many different stories fit this sketch for them all to be neatly squeezed into a simple canonical form. Yet even if the focus on a few key mechanisms might appear dangerously reductive, it has the merit of identifying 'zones of concern' that might require particular attention. Of necessity, our stylized version factors out many important features that have been determinant in certain critical circumstances, but it is comprehensive enough to provide a provisional map allowing us to sort out, in a preliminary way, some of the important sources of potential governance failures. Much that is idiosyncratic to particular cases needs to be added to make sense of the particulars of any specific issue. But the 'simplifying filter' we propose has much to offer as a guide to the inquiry, and much problem-solving power as well.

Loci of pathologies of governance

In the first place, there is a lack of recognition, and even a denial, of the fundamental complexity of our modern socio-technical systems. Jay Forrester (1971) has done significant work that has thrown much light on the dynamics of such systems, and has shown that their behaviour is often counter-intuitive and unpredictable. It often leads unsuspecting observers and experts (insistent on holding to their more simplistic views of the world) to develop strategies and policies, and to minimize some of the negative impacts ensuing from the unconstrained evolution of such systems, by taking action that is, in fact, making things worse. This is mainly because the dynamics of complex, socio-technical systems are poorly understood, unless one is armed with a less inadequate epistemology than the ones in good currency. We refer to the ensuing pathology as **the Forrester effect**.

As Wassily Kandinsky put it, while the 19th century was more an age of 'either-or', the 20th (and *a fortiori* the 21st) century has been (is) an age dominated by 'and': an age of multiplicity, plurality, simultaneity, connections, globalization of side-effects, cumulative causation, and boomerang effects (Beck 1997).

As a result, the dual optimisms of some observers of the past (presuming linear progress with the advent of modernity and scientization, generating ever more effective controllability of the side-effects generated by the heightened interdependencies) have been starkly contradicted by historical experience. More and more we find ourselves, as Beck suggests, "in situations which the prevailing institutions and concepts of politics can neither grasp nor adequately respond to" (*Ibid.*: 7).

Two of the key features of Beck's diagnosis on the sort of modernity we are experiencing are that (1) modern societies "largely produce of their own accord the problems and challenges which confront them" (*Ibid.*: 40), that they have become manufacturers of danger, and that one can no longer ascribe the source of these dangers to external causes; and (2) science becomes more and more necessary but less and less sufficient for ascertaining the nature of these dangers, and for remedying the problems they entail (Beck 2003: 343ff). This is **the Beck effect**.

Both citizens and the media have failed to understand that decisions in the face of high uncertainty are, of course, subject to error. So when such errors or misfortunes occur, they slip easily into fear and outrage, and become obsessed with finding individual adversaries or outside institutions to carry the blame.

What ensues is a complacent wallowing in 'a culture of entitlement to absolute protection' from unpleasant outcomes. One hundred percent protection from bad outcomes is both desired and seen as mandatory. The citizenry has proved quite unwilling either to take stock of the complexity of the situations, or to appreciate the limitations on effective action when concerns about the danger factors can only be poorly characterized from a scientific point of view (May 1994).

This lack of critical thinking is ascribable in part to the great complexity of the issues, to the carelessness and biases of the media coverage, and also to the culture of our modern industrial societies: a culture of blaming, "ready to treat every death as chargeable to someone's account, every accident as caused by someone's criminal negligence" (Douglas 1992: 15) – **the Douglas effect.**

In the modern contexts where power, resources and information are widely distributed, collective action is required to resolve issues of interest. This often commands collaboration by persons or groups in conflictive equilibrium – none of them being in charge, nor able to get rid of their competitors – indeed, needing them as collaborators to resolve issues to their benefit, but hesitant to enter into such collaboration. This is because collaboration is not easily achieved unless it is understood as requiring a new relationship that is characterized by mutuality and respect (devoid of paternalism), and entails genuine co-production of collective decisions and services. Such a new relationship must be based on trust, and fails miserably when influenced by a mutual lack of respect by one's partners (Goss 2007).

In the maze of cross-responsibilities in the blood transfusion system, for instance, (with its political-bureaucratic interface, the tension between science-based and medical personnel, and the parochial mentality of so many provincial public sector representatives), collaboration and partnering can be immensely difficult and fraught with blockages – **the Goss effect.** This is especially destructive when friction among technocrats of different lineages allows the main purpose of the collective action to be lost sight of, and when the uneasy partnership constitutes a monopoly not blessed with enough competition to keep it honest.

In the face of (1) incomplete information and knowledge about these complex, socio-technical systems, (2) imperfect coordination because power, resources and information were widely distributed, and (3) learning disabilities ascribable to the very difficulty of getting reluctant partners to work in synchrony – mishaps have occurred that cannot reasonably be ascribed to a person or a group, but instead to the insurmountable imperfections of continually evolving systems.

These failures have often been transformed from tragedies into scandals by experts who inflicted unreasonable standards on what they label the 'expected performance of officials': *ex post facto* manufactured expectations that have gone much beyond anything that scientific evidence would warrant *ex ante*.

In some cases, clairvoyance is postulated as not only possible but mandated, and the use of the so-called **precautionary principle** becomes instrumental in criminal negligence being automatically argued whenever an accident occurs. This is the world of 'you ought to have known.' The whole world of governance failures is therefore transformed by a sleight of hand. Effective governance ceases to be gauged on the basis of a fair assessment of the *ex ante*, existing state of knowledge and evidence, but by reference to an *ex post facto*, defined yet unreasonable standard of clairvoyance.

Whether or not there has been a governance failure in such a complex context, it has often come to require a particularly careful *ex post* expert analysis. This has led to the creation of commissions of inquiry of all sorts, charged with a careful analysis of the circumstances of the different cases in point. Much that surrounds this process of adjudication has been questionable: the nature of the mandate, the standards of admissible evidence, the ceremonials and etiquette observed, and the place allowed for emotional, but baseless rants and denunciations. Indeed, the general quality of such adjudication has been rather low by the standards defined by ordinary courts.

This has often meant that persons or groups have been singled out as deserving to be investigated further, and brought to court (or have been led to plea bargain to avoid such proceedings threatening to last for years) on the basis of the flimsiest of evidence. A fair number of cases predicated on such 'evidence' have been thrown out of court in the recent past.

One might reasonably have hoped that the police investigations triggered by the flimsy evidence gathered by petulant or incompetent commissions of inquiry would be quickly terminated, if it turned out that the commission was carried away by forces that had nothing to do with substantive proof of guilt. However, this is not always so. Once the process of investigation is launched, the 'cascading logic' of the commission of inquiry, of the police investigation that often ensues, and of the offices of attorneys general brought into the file, often develops into **a logic of indictment seeking**.

This leads commissions of inquiry, police forces and the Office of an Attorney General (wittingly or not) to develop a 'mindset focused on getting an indictment', rather than (1) establishing the facts clearly and independently, and (2) determining whether the uncovered facts, in their totality, warrant an indictment to be brought forth.

The sheer determination to get an indictment has led to testimonies being suppressed, and selective inattention being given to evidence raising fundamental questions about culpability. This would appear to be less a case of individual malice than the result of 'a culture of success' – being defined as getting an indictment. Such mishaps are often corrected by official courts of law – a locus where the standards of evidence are less whimsical. But such court decisions often come years after the original investigation, and the exoneration receives nothing like the attention in the media that the inquiry and the original indictment got. As a result, the shadow of guilt is never quite lifted from the head of the falsely-accused, and the process of social learning (that would call for an organizational redesign to ensure that the misfortune or accident that triggered the whole affair will be much less likely in the future) gets derailed.

Pathological cascade

The different mechanisms (the Forrester effect, the Beck effect, the Douglas effect, the Goss effect, the precautionary principle as the new guidepost, and the logic of indictment seeking) mentioned in the last section are not always instrumental or operative in the genesis of all disastrous episodes.

For all sorts of reasons, many or all of these pathologies may be inoperative in a given file: the relevant uncertainty and the dynamics of the socio-technical system may be fully and effectively factored in; collaboration may blossom; actors may be unusually clairvoyant and lucky, etc. In such cases, there is no mistake or error, and interventions (when necessary) are effective and take fully into account all the side-effects. Citizens and media resist the urge to indict. Adjudication and police investigations proceed with propriety, care and wisdom, and in a perfectly sensible and balanced way.

However, the obverse occurs too often: the complex system not being fully understood and controllable, errors occur; citizens, media and lobby groups whip up a storm, and the adjudication process and police investigations can be derailed by such social movements into generating flawed results. So the possibility of many slippages along the way can clearly not be ruled out.

The tainted-blood tragedy as a cascade of governance failures

In the case studied in this book, it would appear, on the basis of a provisional examination of the issue domain, that:

1. all these mechanisms may have come into play;
2. their cumulative impact may have generated an unnecessary ordeal for many persons; and
3. little or no social learning would appear to have taken place about the ways in which the public health system (or other complex, socio-technical systems likely to be subjected to unthinkable shocks – like public safety) should be redesigned to minimize the damages likely to ensue.

Many questions remain, of which the following are only a few:

How inadequate was the appreciation of the complexity of the issues in 1982 when the AIDS epidemic struck?

How has the lack of effective coordination among the different stakeholders contributed to this systemic muddle?

How flawed have the processes of inquiry and investigation been?

What lessons can be learned from what has been experienced in the handling of this accident to the blood distribution system in Canada?

Are there better ways to deal with the blame equation in our high-risk society?

What role should the precautionary principle be allowed to play (and not allowed to play) if it is not to challenge the crucial democratic principle of the presumption of innocence?

What fail-safe mechanisms may be required to ensure that we can do better next time there is a challenge of the sort that the AIDS epidemic has generated?

These are some of the questions that the book will try to answer.

The dynamics of harm

To proceed usefully with any sort of inquiry such as our own, it is necessary to be aware of the great difference between the 'evasive thinking' usually underpinning the efforts to promote good things, and the sort of 'intellectual work' usually required to reduce or limit bad things. On the surface, they may look the same, but, at the operational level, it makes a considerable difference: "scrutinizing the harms themselves, and discovering their dynamics and dependencies, leads to the possibility of sabotage. Cleverly conceived acts of sabotage, exploiting identified vulnerabilities of the object under attack, can be not only effective, but extremely resource-efficient too" (Sparrow 2008: 27). Any meaningful study must aim at uncovering the dynamics of harms in the way complex, socio-technical systems react to unforeseeable shocks, in order to be able to suggest ways to 'sabotage' the process that generates ineffective and unfair outcomes.

Only through a careful description can one hope to reconstruct the blood transfusion system as a dynamic open-ended process (that is interfered with by external surprises, and a plurality of actors attempting to change it to fit their priorities), to understand the intricacies of the points in contention, and what is required to ascertain whether the actions taken were reasonable and prudent, or not. These are the matters on which the stylized process of indictment rests or fails.

It is too simple to ascribe all failures to malevolent external surprises. Complex, socio-technical systems are also subjected to internal pressures emerging from the gradual uncovering of the different stakeholders' intentions, projects and power moves, from critiquing them, and acting upon lessons learned (Jessop 2003: 7). To probe at this level requires 'reconstructive work' around some crucial contentious issues (1) to show the limitations of the particular reconstructions that both Justice Krever and the RCMP would appear to have conceived, (2) the reasons why their representations may have been flawed, and, as a matter of consequence, (3) what may have led to a decision to indict that proved widely off the mark.

Any reconstructive work of this sort is not unlike the inquiry referred to in Arturo Pérez-Reverte's novel *The Flanders Panel*, in which the action pivots around a painting of a nobleman and a chevalier playing a game of chess. The painter is said to have painted it two years after the death of the chevalier, and has inscribed on the painting the cryptic statement 'who has taken the knight?' that might also have meant 'who has killed the chevalier?' A restoration artist obtains the help of a skilled chess player to reconstruct the game and to discover who has taken the knight. The expert proceeds in this difficult reconstruction, starting from the end situation on the chessboard and working backward through the earlier possible moves, eliminating the impossible moves, and arriving logically at the conclusion that the last move was played by the black queen. This is the genius of reconstruction: to start with the end structure to recreate the process that has resulted in this structure, so as to gain *"une compréhension proprement historique de la situation donnée"* (Ferry 1996: 9ff).

The basic argument in brief and provisionally

The basic argument that our book wishes to put to a test is that the tainted-blood tragedy was a cascade of governance failures, best summarized in very stark terms as follows:

Context

An entirely new virus (the source and dissemination process of which was poorly understood, even though it had been incubating for several years) hit a blood transfusion system that was ill-equipped to respond quickly because of its many flawed features:

1. its monopoly situation made it less than fully sensitive to the evolving context;
2. an inter-provincial administrative structure made its funding dependent on an acrimonious, antagonistic and excessively myopic mentality of provincial bureaucrats;
3. an awkward management structure prevented quick decision making in the face of critical new developments; and
4. a fragmented and non-collaborative *ethos* existed in a multi-stakeholder governing structure.

Reactive capability

This entailed a reactive and rather conservative governance style that did not allow bold pre-emptive moves, but rather only very slow, painful action unsuited for crisis management. So as the crisis unfolded, the incapacity of the routine maladaptive management structure to shift to a crisis and risk management mode, and the extraordinarily uncooperative spirit inhabiting the interprovincial arrangements proved lethal.

A perfect storm

However imperfect the reaction of the system to the crisis, the unwillingness of the provinces, *ex post*, to accept a no-fault compensation scheme fuelled a blaming game that was fed by:

1. a vociferous lobbying process of the group hardest hit by the AIDS epidemic – the hemophiliacs;

2. the uncritical and inflammatory coverage of the evolving issue by the media;
3. this put pressure on the politicians, ensuring that emotions inhabited both the experience of the crisis and the whole investigation in the aftermath;
4. the drive to find and expose culpable parties which took hold of the investigation (at the inquiry level, at the police work level, and at the Attorney General level) and became a substitute for appropriate governance risk repairs; and
5. the broad scoping of the issue by Justice Krever, the police work to determine the facts, and the appraisal work by the Attorney General's Office about the evidence accumulated became confounded into a single drive to indict.

Little was learned about the basic causes of the tragedy, and therefore the 'governance regime' that has ensued would appear not to be as well prepared as it should for the next crisis.

In summary

The whole experience could have generated much social learning if more mindfulness had been mustered in the analysis of the whole affair, for much was evident:

1. about the poor inter-provincial capacity to cooperate even in matters of life or death;
2. about the poor capacity to react effectively and collaboratively to unthinkable events unless some emergency preparedness apparatus is ready to kick in;
3. about the unlikelihood that the interest groups, the media and the political officials might react with anything but emotional outbursts unless expert critical situation networks could be activated to temporarily contain the emotional drive and steward the collective action in useful directions;
4. about the fact that one could not count on the sort of quasi-judicial commissions of inquiry, police investigation, or the provincial governments' legal apparatus to provide a fair-minded process of evaluation of the governance

system failures *ex post* (and therefore to suggest effective repairs) when encapsulated in the *ethos* following tragedies of that sort;

5. about the propensity to ascribe governance failures to a person or persons, at each of these stages of the evolution of the crisis, and to indict officials' failure to live up to their burden of office as the cause of the tragedy;

6. about the recognition that only a formal examination by a court of law would appear equipped to correct these *dérapages* upstream, and yet this is a process that was both extremely late in coming, and so costly as to lead to a denial of justice for many who were wronged in the process; and

7. about the need for major repairs to be effected to much of the apparatus in place to enable it to deal with the next crisis; otherwise, the probability of governance failures, and of miscarriage of justice will remain very high.

Provisional conclusion

Any organization is built on the assumption that those who choose to become associates have a will to engage and to contribute actively to the common work. In French law, this sort of spirit of collaboration has a name – *affectio societatis*. It is a most important element in corporate law, more or less capturing the fact that partners enter into a partnership in good faith, with a will to associate, and a commitment that is consequential (Cuisinier 2008). In French law, failure to demonstrate *affectio societatis* may lead to the dissolution of the partnership.

Evidence of a lack of *affectio societatis* seems obvious when probing the tainted-blood tragedy file. Yet it is a constitutive element of organizations. An active and creative contribution to the association or partnership is expected, is part of a postulated moral contract, and therefore is part of the burden of office of the associates. A delinquent associate (i.e., one failing to provide *affectio societatis*) is in breach of contract, and fails to live up to his burden of office. Consequently, shirking in such circumstances is not only the source of inefficiency, but a form of disloyalty that is quite consequential.

Yet one of the most extraordinarily important missing characteristics in most organizations or regimes or systems, is the 'commitment to collaborate in order to succeed'. Incentive reward systems may help resolve part of this problem, but it cannot be done well without being complemented by moral contracts, if effective performance is to be generated (Paquet and Ragan 2012). Consequently, governance repairs most often require not only architectural modifications, but also an enrichment of the regime of engagement by moral contracts and intersubjective structures (Fullbrook 2002; Thévenot 2006).

This triggers new imperatives when considering organizational repairs.

First, it underlines the fact that disloyalty may be the result not only of acts of commission but also of acts of omission. This is similar to failure to provide help to persons in difficulties at an accident scene, or failure to provide professional defense to employees that are regarded as reprehensible. Second, it dramatically illustrates the fact that failure of engagement and commitment may be a form of disloyalty. Finally, it suggests that the burden of office as a nexus of moral contracts may be difficult to define, but that its very existence is at the core of the effectiveness of organizations (Paquet 2010).

One cannot mandate commitment and loyalty, but there are ways to improve the conditions allowing such sentiments to emerge and to nudge them into existence. The road to collaborative governance is therefore long and arduous (Paquet 2009). As to the design of such pre-conditions for success, some templates exist to match the spans of control (hard) and influence (soft) so as to meet the span of accountability (hard) and support (soft) (Simons 2005).

In such matters, scheming virtuously is not an option ... it is the only way.

References

Beck, Ulrich. 1997. *The Reinvention of Politics*. Cambridge, UK: Polity Press.

Beck, Ulrich. 2003. *La société du risqué*. Paris, FR: Flammarion.

Cuisinier, Vincent. 2008. *L'affectio societatis*. Paris, FR: Litec.

Douglas, Mary. 1992. *Risk and Blame*. London, UK: Routledge.

Ferry, Jean-Marc. 1996. *L'éthique reconstructive*. Paris, FR: Les Éditions du Cerf.

Forrester, Jay W. 1971. "Counterintuitive Behavior of Social Systems," *Technology Review*, 73(3): 52-68.

Fullbrook, Edward (ed.). 2002. *Intersubjectivity in Economics*. London, UK: Routledge.

Gawande, Atul. 2009. *The Checklist Manifesto – How to get things right*. New York, NY: Metropolitan Books.

Goss, Sue. 2007. "How far have we traveled towards a collaborative state?" in S. Parker and N. Gallagher (eds.). *The Collaborative State*. London, UK: Demos, p. 38-47.

Hubbard, Ruth and Gilles Paquet. 2007. *Gomery's Blinders and Canadian Federalism*. Ottawa, ON: The University of Ottawa Press.

Jessop, Bob. 2003. *Governance and Meta-governance: On Reflexivity, Requisite Variety and Requisite Irony*, http://comp.;ancs.ac.uk/sociology/soc108rj.htm.

May, Peter J. 1994. "A Dialogue about Risk," *Journal of Contingencies and Crisis Management*, 2(3): 174-178.

O'Neill, Onora. 2002. *A Question of Trust*. Cambridge, UK: Cambridge University Press.

Paquet, Gilles. 2009. *Scheming Virtuously: The Road to Collaborative Governance*. Ottawa, ON: Invenire Books.

Paquet, Gilles. 2010. "Disloyalty," *www.optimumonline.ca*, 40(1): 23-47.

Paquet, Gilles and Tim Ragan. 2012. *Through the Detox Prism: Exploring Organizational Failures and Design Responses*. Ottawa, ON: Invenire Books.

Simons, Robert. 2005. *Levers of Organization Design*. Boston, MA: Harvard Business School Press.

Sparrow, Malcolm K. 2008. *The Character of Harms*. Cambridge, UK: Cambridge University Press.

Thévenot, Laurent. 2006. *L'action au pluriel – Sociologie des régimes d'engagement*. Paris, FR: Éditions La Découverte.

CHAPTER 2

| Four Ill-founded Accusations

Introduction

T his second chapter deals with the four areas of purported failure by the Canadian Red Cross (and other parties), identified in a letter by the Canadian Hemophilia Society (CHS) to the RCMP, immediately after the report of Justice Krever's inquiry on the tainted-blood tragedy was tabled. These four accusations, articulated by the CHS and based on its interpretation of the findings of the Krever Commission, became canonical: they were widely disseminated in the popular press; they were the foundation on which the presumption of guilt of the Canadian Red Cross was constructed in the media; and they were the basis for the initiation of court proceedings against Dr. Perrault and other parties later on.

The general formulation of these four accusations has been as follows:

The decision not to introduce surrogate testing for the hepatitis C virus between 1986 and 1990.

In his report, Judge Krever said that this failure led to the infection of 28,000 Canadians, and that 85% of those cases were preventable.

Delays in introducing testing for HIV in the blood supply.

A test was available on March 2, 1985, but universal testing was not put in place until November 1 of that year. The report concluded that at least 133 people contracted the AIDS virus in that period.

Delays in the introduction of concentrates that were heat-treated. *A decision was made in November 1984 to switch to the safer product, but it was not completed until July 1985. Judge Krever concluded that the inventory of unheated products was deliberately exhausted and, had blood system officials acted promptly, "some of the hemophiliacs would have avoided being infected."*

Continued use of heat-treated products, as late as 1987, after this method had been proved ineffective. *After the belated switch to heat-treated concentrate, questions remained about the efficacy of heating methods to kill the virus; that, coupled with the fact that manufacturers continued to use plasma that was not tested for the AIDS virus, led to the infection of a number of other hemophiliacs in 1986-87, after the products were declared free of HIV."*

This second chapter intends to show in Part I that these accusations about reprehensible delays, ascribable to the negligence of the Canadian Red Cross (CRC), were groundless. In Part II, we show that such unwarranted accusations were meant to be brought to court by the Crown – although the first three were withdrawn after the fourth one had been adjudicated by Justice Benotto in October 2007. The withdrawal of the charges was the result of shoddy investigative work, and of a 'logic of indictment seeking whatever' fed by the 'precautionary principle' and a process totally unchallenged by 'yellow' journalism.

PART I.
The groundlessness of the four accusations

Accusation no. 1

The decision not to introduce surrogate testing for the hepatitis C virus between 1986 and 1990.

In his report, Judge Krever said that this failure led to the infection of 28,000 Canadians, and that 85% of those cases were preventable.

Nature of the problem

Before 1989, the viruses at the source of hepatitis A and B were known, and carriers of the virus could be screened out of the flow of blood donors. It was also known that another source of hepatitis existed, one that could not be ascribed to the known viruses (A and B). It was this other form of hepatitis (non-A and non-B) which materialized and infected blood recipients.

A surrogate test was used in certain countries to eliminate from the flow of potential donors those with high levels of the enzyme ALT in their blood. Certain experts felt that this surrogate test suggested the presence of an infectious agent that might be the source of hepatitis, non-A and non-B. The so-called surrogate test was known as a marker of liver dysfunction.

In the US, one major study by the National Heart, Lung and Blood Institute (Aach *et al.* 1981) seemed to favour, on balance, the use of this test to screen blood donors. However, this was not universally accepted. A second study, carried out by the National Institutes of Health (Alter *et al.* 1981), did not recommend the use of the ALT-based surrogate test. The American Red Cross (AmCross), in its own study of February 1985 (quoted in Krever 1997, vol 2: 634), found that ALT levels varied widely depending on geography, alcohol use, and even blood types. It concluded that "ALT testing raises more questions than it answers." The American Association of Blood Banks (AABB) felt that definitive prospective studies were required before introducing ALT testing (October 1985), as quoted in Krever 1997 (vol 2: 636).

Although the efficacy of the surrogate test remained unproven, this test became part of common practice in the United States as a result of the pressure of competition in the market among the many companies supplying blood products. This surrogate test screening came to be seen as an additional, though unproven, safeguard. Such a safeguard was valued by some customers, so they were willing to pay for it in a system where blood was supplied on a cost recovery basis. In Canada, blood was provided free of charge to hospitals for the use of the patients, and paid for by the provincial governments, which were not ready to pay for an unproven test.

Between 1986 and 1990, this surrogate test was used neither in Canada nor in the UK (where a single national supplier also existed). Indeed, the blood banking community was opposed to using a surrogate test.

Rationale for not using the surrogate test

The rationale for not using the surrogate test in Canada was simple. Its efficacy was regarded by experts as unproven and, therefore, it was difficult for the Canadian Red Cross (CRC) to make a case for funding from the Canadian Blood Committee (CBC) – and through it from the provincial governments – to implement the use of this surrogate test.

It should be understood that the relationship between the CRC and the CBC was tense. The blood system was becoming more and more sophisticated, and therefore more and more costly, and the CBC was drawing the funding for the blood system from the overall funding that had been approved by the provincial governments for their hospitals. Any additional expense that the CRC wanted to have authorized was contentious, for it meant denying access to money for other hospital services. So the burden of proof was on the CRC to show that it was essential.

In such matters, the point of view of the experts at the LCDC (Laboratory Centre for Disease Control), (or its Bureau of Biologics) was obviously most important. Since the efficacy of the test remained unproven, it is easy to understand that the Bureau of Biologics or the CBC might hesitate to order the use of such a test. The fact that the Bureau of Biologics did not demand that the surrogate test be used (or even stated that it was essential) played a key role. Without such an order or a very strong recommendation, there would be resistance on the part of the province-based committee charged with the funding responsibilities for the blood system to approve the funding for such a test and allow other hospital costs to remain unfunded.[1]

---

[1] Such a surrogate test would entail important costs to implement it, but since the test was imperfect, it would generate many false positives, and consequently important follow-up costs for those patients who, even though they had no sign of infection, would have to be subjected to extensive subsequent testing and care.

Accusation no. 2

Delays in introducing testing for HIV in the blood supply. A test was available on March 2, 1985, but universal testing was not in place until November 1 of that year. The report concluded that at least 133 people contracted the AIDS virus in that period.

It is true that a test to screen blood donors for HIV was made commercially available in March 1985, and testing began in the next few weeks across all systems in the US. In Canada, testing began only in August 1985 – with complete implementation of the test on a national scale at all the blood centres in Canada on November 1, 1985 – something that was not yet in place even in the United States.

This latter date (which has too often been wrongly quoted as the beginning date of testing, when, in fact, it was the moment when national testing was in place, coast-to-coast) has been a major source of disinformation during the whole period of the tainted-blood tragedy in Canada. But it is nevertheless clear that there was a delay between the time testing started in the US and when it started in Canada. This was ascribable to the differences in the nature of the blood systems.

Nature of the problem

Canada had a national blood system, whereas the American blood system was made up of a multiplicity of independent groups – AmCross, Council of Community Blood Centres (CCBC), United Blood Services, and AABB (American Association of Blood Banks) which regrouped several small individual blood banks – all groups working *without* the heavy administrative structure and regimen imposed on the National Blood System in Canada.

The component groups of the US systems worked in competition with one another. They had an incentive to adjust to new circumstances as rapidly as possible in order not to lose market share to more agile competitors. Portions of this decentralized and polymorphous US system, operating on a cost-recovery basis with their hospital clients, could take action immediately, as soon as the test became available. This was bound to be faster than the highly and strictly financially controlled Canadian National Blood System (CNBS). The CNBS could not take action unless it had the authorization and funding from the Canadian Blood Committee (CBC) – a federal-provincial committee that required the agreement of the different provinces – an agreement that could emerge only after a labourious and lengthy process in most circumstances.

The process at work was in two stages, involving the decision to proceed and the implementation. First, the decision to proceed is one taken by the CBC. In this case, the CBC did not get an agreement from all provinces easily.

Two provinces (Ontario and Manitoba) held up a decision for a while. Second, to get authorization to proceed with the initiation of testing in Canada, there was the need to prepare an implementation plan for the National Advisory Committee on AIDS (NACAIDS) (done by May 1, 1985). This required plans for staff training, for testing set up, for evaluation of the various kits and, finally, for the approval of the kits by the Bureau of Medical Devices (BMD) of Health and Welfare Canada.

Formal approval to begin testing was received by the Canadian Red Cross Blood Transfusion Service (BTS) on August 1, 1985. Testing began within the same month in some blood centres, where minimal alterations to the laboratories were needed. In other more "dated" centres, the process took more time. By November 1,. 1985, testing was in place across the whole Canadian system, and hospitals had refreshed their stock with HIV-tested blood.

Commentary

The vast majority of countries have more or less independent regional transfusion centres. Therefore, national data about the moment when full coverage at the national level was in place was difficult to obtain or to verify. So it is important to be suspicious of some international comparisons in such cases, for most of the time it is unknown exactly and really when the implementation of a test had been completed and could claim to be nationally in place.

In the case of Canada – with its full national system – we know that the complete national testing was in place coast-to-coast by November 1, 1985. Where a large number of independent suppliers were in place, it has remained problematic to make such a statement. However, all through the period of the blood tragedy, very many uninformed and unreliable statements about foreign, decentralized schemes were merrily quoted to damn the Canadian situation, without any credible sources to back them up.

Accusation no. 3

Delays in the introduction of concentrates that were heat-treated. A decision was made in November 1984 to switch to the safer product, but it was not completed until July 1985. Justice Krever concluded that the inventory of unheated products was deliberately exhausted and, had blood system officials acted promptly, "some of the hemophiliacs would have avoided being infected" [our underlining].

The nature of the problem

Following the AIDS outbreak in 1982, heat-treated concentrates to kill the HIV virus were developed by large plasma fractionators in the industrialized countries.

These developments were consequential:

- loss of product (approx. 20 percent) of this very labile protein molecule, due to the heating process;
- level of viral kill: each company developed its own process aimed at achieving the highest possible "kill" level, while minimizing the loss of product in the process;
- availability of product from the large manufacturers that were attempting to meet demand from customers worldwide, keeping in mind the 20 percent loss to the overall world supply;
- rate of introduction of the new product as it became available: i.e., who gets first call on the available product, when it arrives in unpredictable quantities;
- withdrawal of the untreated concentrates; and
- additional testing by the Bureau of Medical Devices (BMD), Health and Welfare Canada.

At the December 10, 1984 Consensus Conference, the interested parties[2] addressed the above issues.

It is essential to first eliminate the red herrings if one is to understand what went on:

- The provinces had agreed to pay for this new and very expensive product.
- The CBC had agreed to pay for all the unused unheated product, when it became aware that some of the heated products were defective because donors had not been properly screened. Therefore, there was no economic incentive for ever using any of the defective product, unless it turned out to be the only alternative material available that patients would accept in the event of shortage of supply of the entirely-safe, heated product.

There was anticipation that the supply of safe, heated products would not meet the demand in the transition period, so the Consensus Conference had agreed that there would be distribution of a mixture of old and new product during the phase-in period.

There were 39 recommendations arising from the conference, and the Canadian Red Cross was asked to implement the recommendations outlined below (nos. 1, 3, 4 and 8):

#1: "That this Conference endorses the introduction of heat-treated Factor VIII concentrates in Canada as soon as is feasible before May 1985, with a transition period not exceeding eight weeks thereafter when both heat-treated and non-heat-treated will be transfused to Canadian hemophiliacs."

[2] Conference participants:
- from CBC: 18 (for the provinces, the Secretariat and the Advisory Committee)
- from Canadian Hemophilia Society: 3
- from fractionation industry: 7
- from Health and Welfare Canada: 2
- from National Advisory Committee on AIDS: 1 (chairman)
- from the Canadian Red Cross BTS: 6

#3: "That this Conference recommends that all Factor VIII products currently in the plasma or cryoprecipitate stages should be heat-treated."

#4: "That this Conference recognizes that the CRC will continue to direct all FFP to facilities currently licensed to produce heat-treated Factor VIII until Canadian Fractionators are licensed to produce heat-treated concentrates, when the CRC will redirect plasma to licensed Canadian facilities."

#8: "That this Conference recommends that the criteria for the use of heat-treated and non-heat-treated concentrate during the transition period be agreed upon by the hemophilia treaters who are members of the Medical/ Scientific Advisory Committee of the CHS, using existing national representation."

Implementation of the Consensus Conference decisions
The source of the delay in this instance was that the suppliers could not cope with the burst of demand worldwide.

Keeping in mind the need for securing purchasing capacity with foreign fractionators, who were gearing up to supply the world market (and the difficult position of Canadian fractionators, unlicensed to provide heat-treated Factor VIII concentrate in a timely fashion), the bottleneck was created by both the shortage of supply *and* the reluctance/unwillingness of the hemophiliacs to return to the earlier and much more cumbersome method of treatment with cryoprecipitates (even for a transition period until suppliers could catch up to meet demand for heated products). In this latter case, the reluctance was due to the fact that the old method was immensely inconvenient for the patients.

Why was unheated product used at all?
The choice was unheated product or the treatment with cryoprecipitates. There was a risk in using the unheated product, but given the circumstances, this was a known fact. Hemophiliacs had the choice to go back to the earlier treatment using cryoprecipitates, yet found it unacceptable. At the Consensus Conference (which included representatives from

the Canadian Hemophilia Society), it had been agreed that unheated product could be used during the transition period.

Some confusion may have been generated about the real nature of the shortage of heated products since large companies were hesitant to admit they could not supply every customer at the same time, but their Canadian representatives confirmed that this was a major issue. On the other hand, we know that the Canadian Red Cross was treated well by the suppliers, since it found itself answering requests for assistance from smaller blood centres in the US who were faced with dire shortages for their patients.

All BTS centres were informed of these developments in a memo from Dr. D. Naylor on March 29, 1985.

Undoubtedly, hemophiliacs were inconvenienced, and some were hurt because they did not want to return to cryoprecipitates. Even their officials agreed.

The Canadian Hemophilia Society (CHS) informed Dr. Naylor (the CRC) on April 25, 1985 of its own action on the recommendations of the Consensus Conference: i.e., identifying the "individuals to whom preference is to be given during the conversion period" (Letter from Dr. Robert Card of the CHS to Dr. Derek Naylor of the CRC, April 25, 1985).

Accusation no. 4

Continued use of heat-treated products as late as 1987, after this method had been proved ineffective.

After the belated switch to heat-treated concentrates, questions remained about the efficacy of heating methods to kill the virus; that, coupled with the fact that manufacturers continued to use plasma that was not tested for the AIDS virus, led to the infection of a number of other hemophiliacs in 1986-87, after the products were declared free of HIV."

The nature of the problem
The Armour Co. Factor VIII concentrate claimed to be completely effective in the inactivation of HIV. Yet cases of seroconversions occurred in the UK which coincided with seroconversions in Holland. After an investigation,

it was shown that the Armour product had been prepared from plasma drawn from unscreened donors. As a result, in mid-October 1986, the Canadian Red Cross BTS stopped distribution of Armour heated concentrate prepared from unscreened donors, and (as suggested by the Bureau of Biologics), continued the distribution of donor-screened concentrate. The other products were withdrawn. The CRC-BTS also procured the additional necessary amounts from Cutter and Hyland.

On October 15, 1986, the US FDA held a meeting, confirming the approval of distribution of donor-screened product. The Bureau of Biologics in Canada informed the National BTS that it supported the US action.

Despite these precautions, new seroconversions were reported in BC and Alberta, through an ongoing study of hemophiliacs by Dr. C. Tsoukas in Montreal in 1987. This was reviewed in detail at the Krever Inquiry, and it became the basis for the fourth accusation mentioned in the Canadian Hemophilia Society letter to the RCMP.

The accusation, in this fourth case, was directed to:

- the Armour Pharmaceutical Co. and its Medical Director, Dr. M. Rodell;
- the Bureau of Biologics of National Health and Welfare and its Director, Dr. J. Furesz and his Assistant, Dr. W. Boucher;
- the Canadian Red Cross and Dr. R. Perrault, National Director of the Blood Transfusion Service.

This accusation was the core issue at a trial held in Toronto between February 2006 and June 2007 (judgment by Justice M.L. Benotto on October 1, 2007). The action taken by the CRCS is well covered in the Benotto judgment, p. 38, para 189-191, and reproduced here:

In early to mid October, 1987, Dr. Walker and Mr. Vick learned of seroconversions in Western Camada. They immediately looked into the patient records and began withdrawing all products that the patients had received. On November 7, 1987, Dr. Walker wrote to the BoB announcing the withdrawal (para 189).

Both the CRC and the BoB worked together to share information, track down implicated lots and withdraw them. They were in daily contact. At the time, the seroconversions were not tied to one company and there was a concern about supply as the product was withdrawn (para 190).

In the fall of 1987, the BoB retained Dr. Robert Remis, an epidemiologist and public health specialist. Dr. Remis was told about the cluster of HIV infections among hemophiliac patients in British Columbia. He was asked to carry out an outbreak investigation or field investigation to determine the cause. In connection with this, he travelled to the Kankakee plant with Dr. Boucher. He learned that lots B713308, B71408 and B71508 had all come from the same donor. Dr. Remis testified that this was very important in arriving at an explanation. Soon after, on December 10, 1987 a formal recall of three lots of Armour Factorate was announced by the BoB. They were lots B71308, B71408, and B71508[3] (para 191).

In light of the above information, it became clear that there was no delay created by CRC in these matters. Indeed, Justice Benotto, in her judgment, states on page 63, "the allegation of criminal conduct on the part of these men (Perrault *et al.*) and this corporation were not only unsupported, they were disproved."

The fourth accusation covered an event that was considerably less complex than the other three. It was a likely factor in its choice as the first charge to be prosecuted by the Office of the Attorney General of Ontario. In the second trial, in Hamilton, January 18, 2008, the Crown attorney asked that the three remaining charges be withdrawn as there seemed to be no realistic chance of a conviction.

---

[3] In referring to "that the three lots came from the same donor": one should point out that this meant that the same infected donor had provided plasma to the three mentioned lots.

PART II.
Why were these groundless accusations brought to court?

Let us reiterate that there is no denying that a blood tragedy occurred, and that victims died or were hurt as a consequence. The issue here is not to deny the tragedy, but to question the underlying presumption that seems to have presided over the whole handling of this tragedy: the idea that if there is a tragedy, there must be someone who is responsible for it, and that this *someone* should be held accountable and punished for it. This presumption denies the possibility of any tragedy orphaned of a personalized responsibility – i.e., any possibility of systemic failure and systemic responsibility – and feeds a determination to establish a link between the tragedy and person or persons to be held responsible for it – whatever the circumstances.

This sort of mental prison is significant for it shapes the framework in use when the whole inquiry process to deal with a tragedy is set into motion:

- the focus is *not* on understanding what is going on in order to effect repairs to avoid such a tragedy in the future, but seeking who should be blamed;
- this, in turn, induces a logic of indictment-seeking that distorts the whole inquiry process: it brings certain elements into focus, while blinding people to other so-called extraneous factors because they may throw light on the events, but are not advancing the search for a guilty party. Those extraneous factors are systematically ignored, even though they may be quite revealing.

This 'righter of wrongs' attitude legitimizes all sorts of shoddiness and short-circuiting in the conduct of the inquiry, when it becomes simply an instrument in the process of reaching an indictment.

For instance,

- giving perhaps too much hearing to aggrieved groups (like the hemophiliacs) and allowing their emotional and aggressively denunciatory action as a lobby group to affect the conduct of the inquiry;

• factoring out reference to the real administrative context and its aberrations, and thereby ignoring the possibility of systemic failures outside the responsibility of any key players;

• indulging in a propensity to predicate that one can assume, with hindsight, an extraordinary clairvoyance on the part of expert actors – and since it is presumed that they should have known, it is naturally presumed also that they did indeed know what their actions would entail. Therefore that they can be indicted for the catastrophe that has ensued, and appropriate expiation can be insisted on. All this thinking is often shrouded in the vapors of the precautionary principle in its more radical version (Wildavsky 1995; Ewald *et al.* 2001); and

• leading the police investigation and the evaluation of the case by the Office of the Attorney General to eliminate inconvenient testimonies in order to better support the case for an indictment.

Given this cascade of pathologies of governance, it is not unusual and abnormal that the media, public opinion, and the soft judiciary (all the quasi-judiciary bodies, like commissions of inquiry etc.) turn out to be unduly influenced by, and even to fall prey to, this logic of indictment (especially when the aggressive lobby is allowed to work promiscuously with the commission of inquiry meant to clarify the issue). All this may readily degenerate into a lynching party.

Some may regard the possibility of such a cascade as so unlikely as to verge on the impossible, but even a casual examination of the tainted-blood tragedy file would convince any dispassionate observer that this sort of cascade of pathologies is exactly what occurred in Canada.

Our intention in this section of the chapter is not to reconstruct the details of all the events surrounding the blood tragedy and wrap it in a melodramatic flavour, but rather to present a certain number of observations that would appear to indicate that the scenario hinted at above is far from improbable.

A summary reconstruction with a certain surreal quality

The first idiosyncratic feature in this case is the complexity of the situation, and the poor capability we and our institutions have to deal effectively with such situations. As Pritchett would put it, most of us are not very good at thinking about system problems. We are good at thinking about objects and agents. But in complex adaptive emergent orders, "the system can have outcomes that no agent in the system intended." Evolutionary processes explain why elephants have long trunks. No central planner has designed it. But "when people do think about systems, they tend to extrapolate their expertise in objects and agents. In other words, they tend to anthropomorphize and tell narratives and reason about systems as if a system were an agent" (Pritchett 2013: 140).

To reduce the complex blood governance system to Roger Perrault – as the agent that might be held responsible for this catastrophe – is senseless and can only lead to a futile search that cannot throw light on what generated a system failure.

The second idiosyncratic feature in this case is the aggressiveness, persistence and penetrative power of the lobbying of the Canadian Hemophilia Society (CHS) into the whole inquiry system. As well documented in Michael Orsini's doctoral thesis (2001), the CHS was not an occasional or episodic lobby group, but an organization that has put relentless pressure on public authorities to identify the persons responsible for this tragedy, and to ensure some punishment for them. It pursued this quest with as much determination as it pursued financial compensation for those hemophiliacs that had been infected. This took the form of a well-organized press campaign, insistent representations to the different governments, interventions pressing for a royal commission, but also a constant presence at the Krever Inquiry, and omnipresence in the shadow of the Attorney General at the trial. This has translated into a promiscuous relation of the CHS with the Krever Inquiry, the Crown's operations, and the 'pursuit of justice' in court.

These two features have helped keep the inquiry process into the Canadian blood tragedy focused on the search for a guilty party to blame, and a **logic of indictment seeking** for the inquiry process. This has led to a third idiosyncratic feature of this case: the confounding of very different segments of the inquiry that are meant to remain tightly sealed one from the other – for their separate functions cannot overlap without the inquiry process being tainted.

For instance, the role of journalists is to report, to reveal anomalies; the role of the police force is to prepare as complete a file as possible – which entails a certain degree of discretion; finally, the justice system has to ascertain whether the matter should be brought to court, which entails a great amount of secrecy. When the aggrieved party engages in as much 'interloping' as the CHS did – in organizing press campaigns, intervening politically, getting closely involved with the quasi-judicial and the judicial process by direct contacts with officials, etc. – this pollination activity may well entail a confounding of activities meant to be strictly separated. Since the single-minded objective of the lobby is to get an indictment of putative guilty parties, the very different functions may also be distorted to work in this direction also, however different their official function may be.

While it is difficult to prove to what extent the interference of the CHS lobby has played a determining role in connecting functions that were meant to be tightly separate, circumstantial evidence of the close rapport between the CHS and the officials of the Krever Commission and of the Crown in the Hamilton trial – as anybody present there can testify – can reasonably lead to the suspicion that this interloping has catalyzed indictment-seeking, taking precedence over the more traditional functions of the diverse actors in this case (Paquet 2012).

A not insignificant side-effect of this commingling of roles has been the way in which the media covered this tragedy. A casual look at two books produced about the case by journalists reveals a bias toward indictment running all the way through (McDuff 1995; Picard 1995).

A fourth idiosyncratic feature of the case is the fact that all of the above has generated a *zeitgeist, un esprit,* a general attitude in the population. So public opinion on the blood tragedy has crystallized in a manner that reflected an immense ignorance of the complexity of the circumstances, a tremendous sympathy for the victims, and an unbounded hostility for those purported by the media to have committed that crime. It was an interesting case of what Tocqueville called "social power" – a dominant opinion that, however ill-founded it might be, becomes so prevalent that any criticism of it proves impotent, and even the political power becomes paralyzed (Boudon 2005: 168).

These four idiosyncratic features constructed a perfect storm.

Conclusion

This *zeitgeist* allowed the Canadian tainted-blood tragedy to sink into 'storytelling' for some 25 years. And when the fairy tale in good currency was finally exposed to a real court of law, Roger Perrault and consorts were fully exonerated.

Still, the real story of the governance failures that generated the Canadian blood tragedy has not been told yet.

That will be discussed in the next chapter.

References

Aach, R.D. *et al.* 1981. "Serum Alanine Aminotransferase of Donors in Relation to the Risk of Non-A, Non-B Hepatitis in Recipients – The Transfusion-Transmitted Virus Study," *New England Journal of Medicine,* 304(17): 980-984.

Alter, H.J. *et al.* 1981. "Donor Transaminase and Recipient Hepatitis – Impact on Blood Transfusion Services," *New England Journal of Medicine,* 246(6): 630-634.

Boudon, Raymond. 2005. *Tocqueville aujourd'hui.* Paris, FR: Odile Jacob.

Ewald, François *et al.* 2001. *Le principe de précaution.* Paris, FR: Presses Universitaires de France.

Krever, Horace. 1997. *Commission of Inquiry on the Blood System in Canada, Final Report.* 3 vols. Ottawa, ON: Minister of Supply and Services Canada.

McDuff, Johanne. 1995. *Le sang qui tue.* Montreal, QC: Libre Expression.

Orsini, Michael. 2001. *Blood, Blame, Belonging: HIV, Hepatitis, and the emergence of tainted-blood activism in Canada 1985-2000.* Doctoral thesis submitted to Carleton University, October 19, 2001.

Paquet, Gilles. 2012. "Médias, imprécations et désinformation," *www.optimumonline.ca*, 42(1): 41-18.

Picard, André. 1995. *The Gift of Death.* Toronto, ON: Harper-Collins.

Pritchett, Lant. 2013. *The Rebirth of Education.* Washington, DC: Center for Global Development.

Wildavsky, Aaron. 1995. "Rejecting the Precautionary Principle" in A. Wildavsky. *But is it true? A citizen's guide to environmental, health and safety issues.* Cambridge, MA: Harvard University Press, p. 427-447.

CHAPTER 3

| A Systemic Deconstruction

Introduction

I n chapter 1, we presented, in a very stylized way, the mechanisms at work in modern, complex, socio-technical systems that might explain why irrational responses to mishaps often transform crises into tragedies, tragedies into scandals, and scandals into miscarriages of justice. We argued that this is what happened in the case of the Canadian tainted-blood tragedy.

In chapter 2, we showed that the four accusations levied against Dr. Perrault and colleagues as a result of the Canadian blood tragedy events were ill-founded. Dr. Perrault was fully exonerated by Justice Benotto in 2007 of the fourth charge, and the other three accusations were withdrawn by the Solicitor General of Ontario, as a result of this acquittal. However, this left the whole issue about the responsibility for this tragedy somewhat unresolved.

In this chapter, we aim to propose a systemic explanation of the sources and causes of the Canadian blood tragedy. It builds on a point that we underlined at the end of the second chapter – the fact that social scientists and media analysts are not very good at thinking about systems problems. Because they mostly know about objects and agents, they tend to anthropomorphize and personalize systems problems, and to reason as if a system were an agent. This, we propose, has been at the basis of many miscarriages of justice. We will proceed with a systemic deconstruction of the Canadian tainted-blood tragedy, and we will provide an alternative explanation of the events surrounding this tragedy as not ascribable to individual faults, but rather to a cascade of governance failures.

This deconstruction proceeds in two stages: first, we expose four pathologies of governance, internal to the existing organization of the blood system, that contributed to governance failures; second, we identify four pathologies of governance, external to the blood system *per se* (but plaguing the administrative system in which it was embedded), that contributed much more significantly to amplifying and exacerbating the tragedy by generating significant governance failures in the way in which the Canadian blood crisis was handled by the institutional context. In our estimation, *in toto*, these pathologies have generated a cascade of governance failures that provides the bulk of the explanation for the Canadian blood tragedy.

Toxic internal pathologies

Before World War II, there was no Canadian civilian blood transfusion system. Each hospital was on its own when it came to its blood supply. Given the success of the Canadian Red Cross (CRC) in dealing with the military`s blood supply during the war, the federal government asked the CRC to extend its work by operating a civilian collection service to meet the needs of both military and civilian hospitals (McDonald 2004: 40).

The Canadian Red Cross Blood Transfusion Service (CRC-BTS) provided a free national blood service for a while. However, as demand grew and transfusion medicine became more sophisticated, the CRC could not continue to supply blood and blood products free of charge to all Canadian hospitals. Provincial and federal governments were pressed to provide financial support. Even though the CRC-BTS had a monopoly on the collection and distribution of blood and blood products, gradually, the provincial governments (responsible for hospitals) and the federal government (responsible for the regulation of pharmaceuticals) became more and more involved in the financing and the regulation of blood collection and transfusion. They also became fundamentally involved in the governance of the system. By 1974, the CRC abdicated control "entirely to government" for all practical purposes (*Ibid.*, p. 44). The sort of shared governance responsibility that ensued made intelligent governance rather difficult.

CRC: an imperfect organization with imperfect oversight

The Canadian Red Cross was a complex organization that dealt with a variety of activities including disaster relief, emergency services, water safety services, first aid services, and homemaker services. Despite its social importance, the Blood Program of the CRC was nothing more than one segment of the CRC, and had only one member out of thirty on the CRC Board – a board that therefore did not necessarily have the full expertise to understand the complexity of the blood system.

As part of the constraints imposed on the CRC, as a result of the tutorship of the International Red Cross, it had to be an independent, neutral body, free from government tutelage. Yet, as it became funded and regulated by the provincial and federal governments for its blood collection and distribution, these principles were compromised.

On the one hand, whether the federal government was intimidated by the humanitarian reputation of the CRC, or whether it was simply neglectful in its governance duties, the custodial regulation of the CRC by the federal government agencies was characterized by experts as "benign neglect" (McDonald *dixit*). Even though the CRC asked to be regulated as of 1981, it was not until 1989 that its blood products were. The CRC remained until then solely responsible for the safety and quality assurance of all its operations: collection, testing, processing, storage and distribution of whole blood and its components (*Ibid.*, p. 54).

On the other hand, from the 1980s on, the Canadian Blood Committee (CBC) – federal and provincial representatives – purported to provide a pseudo-governing framework to ensure that the CRC would fulfill its mandate. It exercised a great deal of control on the CRC of a micromanagement sort – being ferociously stingy every time it came to new financial resources for the BTS, since the cost of the Blood Program had to be extracted from a fixed financial envelope for hospital funding. As McDonald concluded, "the Red Cross could not do the job it needed to do under the constraints of the Canadian Blood Committee's often cumbersome processes" (*Ibid.*, p. 71). It was not until 1991 that the CBC was replaced by a supposedly less cumbersome and more effective arrangement – the Canadian Blood Agency.

Federal-provincial quagmire

Even under what seemed to be an improved arrangement with the creation of the Canadian Blood Agency (CBA) in 1991, and the reforms it brought forth, things did not improve.

The structural arrangement between the regulator, operator and funder remained a major source of problems for the blood system. "The Canadian Blood Agency was a creature of the provinces, designed to work on their behalf 'to direct' the Red Cross's blood system from vein to vein (i.e., the recruitment, collection, processing, and distribution of blood and blood products" (*Ibid.*, p. 73). Since the CBA seemed to have been created solely to act as a way to keep costs under control, safety concerns were bound to arise, and it is not surprising that the CRC would balk at the directives it got from the CBA.

The federal regulator was insistent on safety, but had no role in funding. Provincial authorities wanted lower costs, and did not differentiate between policy directions and specific management issues affecting the safety of blood. The CRC was caught in the middle, and unable to extract satisfactory working arrangements.

This may explain why analysts exploring the tainted-blood tragedy found much responsibility to spread around:

"By the time of the tainted blood scandal, there were so many different groups of people involved in the blood system that it was hard to know who was really in charge. The Red Cross bears partial responsibility for this, but the governments have a much greater culpability; they did not set in place appropriate mechanisms for the governance and funding of Canada's blood supply, and relied too much on a private organization for managing the blood system. What mechanisms were in place – the Canadian Blood Committee and the Canadian Blood Agency – were ineffective in providing policy direction to the Red Cross, and unable to act without information and orders from their respective provincial governments.

The provinces and territories did not live up to their responsibility to provide adequate health care when it came to the blood system. They and their representatives did not really understand how to manage the Red Cross's blood program, nor did the representatives have equal power at the boardroom table. The relationships between governments, representatives, and the Red Cross were completely dysfunctional; no one was in charge during the 1970s and 1980s" (Ibid., p. 120-21).

Resistance, delays and sabotage as transaction costs

As one would expect from such flawed arrangements (and the flawed federal-provincial context in which it was forced to operate), the bureaucratic inertia found much traction. Every occasion for the Red Cross bureaucracy to rein in a line of business that was overwhelming the rest of the organization was effectively used; and every occasion for provincial government representatives to exercise their petty power to scrutinize and to impose delays on an organization that claimed independence, while being substantially financed by provincial governments, was also effectively used. Consequently, there was ever more friction in the governance of what could only be regarded as a blood 'non-system'.

Disagreements were often legitimate, but also often a matter of theatrics. For instance, when an effort was made in the latter part of the 1970s to create a federal-provincial group responsible for governing the blood supply, Quebec pulled out of the committee and dealt with the Red Cross on its own terms. It could be concluded that "governments had stopped working together for a common good as they had in the war years and were engaged in direct competition over every tax dollar" (*Ibid.*, p. 60). In fact, inter-provincial squabbles ensured that provinces took over the governance and funding of the blood system, but never took responsibility for it: "there was a combination of politics and neglect at work" (*Ibid.*, p. 60).

The precautionary principle

At the very time when the demand for blood grew exponentially, the costs also grew, and the governance ran amok. The explicitly un-assumed overall responsibility for the blood system tended to be perceived as having to be accepted by default by an enfeebled and extraordinarily constrained CRC. It was left holding the bag – and was later charged by lobby groups, a commission of inquiry, as a result of an RCMP investigation, and by the Solicitor General of Ontario.

This was – in good part as a result of the new rhetoric of the precautionary principle, which emerged in the 1970s, and had become part of the *culture governance* – the sort of amalgam of attitudes, beliefs, conversations and propensities in the culture that distills a greater likelihood of being swayed by certain points of view (Bang 2003).

The precautionary principle, as a form of prudence that suggests that one should carefully gauge the full range of possible futures before making a final decision, is laudable. However, when such an attitude is not only mandated but judiciarized, and when it is open season on experts, who may be faulted for sins of omission (i.e., for having failed to be clairvoyant), it becomes very dangerous (Ewald *et al.* 2001).

Since the 1970s, it has become the new norm in many areas to hold experts criminally responsible for not having been clairvoyant. Indeed, through the activism of lobby groups, like the Canadian Hemophilia Society, this new norm has been propagandized and widely diffused in the media.

The precautionary principle has become part of the arsenal of interest groups, which have argued that not only should responsibility be personalized, but that lack of clairvoyance should be criminally indictable.

In the face of flawed organizations and institutions, and in the presence of irresponsible and opportunistic behaviour by many parties – over and beyond the abnormal degree of friction that one would expect in multi-stakeholder, complex and uncertain circumstances – the utopian gauge suggested by a radical interpretation of the precautionary principle can only act as a catalyst for unreasonableness.

*   *   *

The combination of these four pathologies has created serious challenges for those charged with the management of the blood system. Clearly nobody was fully in charge, the different groups involved were motivated by quite different objectives, many parties were using the blood system as a pawn in other games of their own, and there was much uncertainty and ignorance in circumstances that were evolving dramatically in real time. Coordination failed, and collaboration was at no time the order of the day. Consequently, it was not surprising that this aggregation of imperfect arrangements generated friction, resistance, and delays, and that these toxic arrangements would ultimately prove lethal.

However, one major player in the psychodrama that ensued as a result of the tragedy has contributed to aggravating the situation, both in the immediacy of the crisis, and in the way in which the follow-up was derailed. The Canadian Hemophilia Society's (CHS) determination to ascribe responsibility for the tragedy to persons – a determination emboldened by the immense difficulty in getting the provincial governments to agree to satisfactory financial compensation for the victims of this tragedy – underpinned understandable but relentless lobbying activities at first. Later, this led to various forms of intervention of a more questionable sort that succeeded in feeding a 'swelling movement' that may be said to have

generated a perfect storm. This was chronicled by Michael
Orsini (2001, 2002).

Venomous external pathologies

The whole apparatus of Canadian institutions charged with
handling crises and governance failures might have been
expected to react to the tainted-blood tragedy by reasonably
ascertaining the sources and causes of the tragedy, avoiding
unwarranted accusations and indictments, and working hard
to reveal the failures in the governing apparatus that might
have caused such tragedy. More satisfactory arrangements
might then have been proposed and put in place. But this was
not to be.

The never-ending lobbying of the CHS
The aggressive and very often misguided lobbying of the CHS
succeeded, with the complicity of the media, in arousing a burst
of sentimentality, grief, and guilt in the population. Moreover,
it benefited from the complicity of provincial governments
in allowing the scapegoating of the CRC and the federal
regulators for the tragedy. For the provincial governments, this
was not an innocent move. It served to deflect attention from
the possibility of any responsibility being ascribed to them in
this whole affair. Consequently, a sort of unwarranted implicit
consensus emerged in the allocation of blame in the whole
affair, and fueled a relentless pursuit of personal indictments of
those scapegoated for the tragedy.

Orsini has thoroughly chronicled the determinant impact
of the CHS's action in all this for the early period.[4] However,
the echo effect of this perfect storm in the latter stages of the
tragedy cycle has not received full attention. More importantly,
perhaps, is the failure to notice that the CHS was the agent that
kept the 'movement' alive all along. At each stage, it ensured
that relentless pressure would continue to be exercised to

[4] Even academic studies like Orsini's doctoral thesis would appear to have been
swayed by the perfect storm: nobody from the CRC-BTS was interviewed as
part of his doctoral study.

ensure that the pursuit of a criminal indictment of particular persons or groups, which the CHS regarded as responsible for the tragedy, would be kept alive. This action received support from the media which transformed this lobbying activity into *pouvoir social* in the sense Tocqueville uses the term.[5] A gauge of the strength of the *pouvoir social* wave that carried public opinion in the 1990s is palpable when one reads two of the books (one in English, and the other in French) that were produced by journalists in 1995 (McDuff 1995; Picard 1995). The cumulative pressure fuelled by the CHS became such that the government felt it could not resist the demand for a commission of inquiry.

The hesitation of the Krever Commission

The CHS was at the forefront of the demand for a commission of inquiry when it realized that negotiations would not yield satisfactory results in terms of compensation for the victims by the provinces. And indeed, because of the social climate at the time, the CHS's demand got the support of many groups that felt that they might benefit from it – in particular, the provinces, which wanted to escape the possibility of any responsibility being directed at them, and were determined to wrestle away from the embrace of the CRC the blood system they were financing.

The CHS and several of its members were given official standing and sustaining funding by the Krever inquiry, and were clearly very influential in the inquiry process.

The nature of a commission of inquiry is to act as a fact finder. However, in this task, it does not operate with the strict procedures of a court of law. The consequence is that what is regarded as acceptable evidence in a commission is often evidence that would be rejected by a court of law. The inquiry

---

[5] Raymond Boudon, a Tocqueville expert, defines *pouvoir social* as *"l'ensemble des relais qui imposent sur tel ou tel sujet une opinion dominante devant laquelle le pouvoir politique se sent comme paralysé ou qu'il doit du moins tenir pour un paramètre essentiel de son action; devant laquelle la critique est par ailleurs impuissante, voire plus ou moins discrètement censurée"* (Raymond Boudon 2005: 168).

received testimonies with a great variation in credibility, and suffered from all the flaws that plague such inquiries (Hubbard and Paquet 2007; Livermore 2010). In the case of the Krever Commission, it is well known that at least one advisor to the commission resigned because of his unease about the commission's approach. Whether it was because of the influence of the CHS is not clear, but the promiscuity of the CHS (which was clearly on a lynching mission) with the commission has been mentioned.

Given the societal pressure on Krever (not only from the CHS but from the whole social movement it initiated), it must be said that the inquiry did a creditable job on many fronts. It brought forth many important dimensions of this complex issue, and did not indict the persons and groups targeted by the lobbyists, although it did not exonerate them either.

Krever's hesitation to clear the names of those targeted by the lobbyists may be explained by his prudence in interpreting his mandate, but it might also be understood as a result of the general *zeitgeist* of the day that would have accepted, with great difficulty, a report that would exonerate, on the basis of the commission's findings. This hesitation left the door open for a continuation of the fight for the CHS.

Other commissions have gone very much further in ensuring that certain parties would be *de facto* immunized from further action, if not officially exonerated. It is not clear why certain parties that were shown to be unjustly targeted by the immense amount of information sifted by the commission, could not legitimately expect that the commission would feel compelled by the complement of evidence it had accumulated to act in a manner that might suppress the odium of additional harassment when the factum would appear to show that those persons were unreasonably targeted.

Determining who should be brought to court

The Krever Commission's sin of omission was consequential. As soon as the Krever Commission tabled its report – in which personal accusations and indictments were *not* suggested, but no one was completely exonerated either – the CHS sent a letter to the RCMP demanding that police action be initiated to ensure that those persons or groups (that the CHS deemed guilty) should be indicted for the four accusations discussed in chapter 2. It would take some additional 14 years (from 1993 to 2007) before a real court of law would exonerate those parties that had been targeted by the CHS.

The RCMP responded with a thorough inquiry that lasted some five years, involved some 15 officers, 700 interviews, two million documents seized, and visits to several countries. Four Crown counsels also worked full time with the squad.

While this investigation was thorough, it did not unfold in a social vacuum. The relentless pressure of the CHS had elicited much sympathy for the victims in the media and in the population at large. While it is difficult to incontrovertibly establish the impact of this *zeitgeist*, or how the pressure for an indictment might have played out in the police inquiry, it would be surprising if it had been zero.

In the same way, the presence of members of the Crown counsel crew working full-time in the squad may appear incestuous. The police inquiry is supposed to establish whether there is any evidence that some indictable act has been committed. Given the dramatic shadow of the victims, the relentless lobby of the CHS over the police inquiry, and the strong sentiment expressed in the media, it would seem to have been imperative to reinforce the wall between the officials of the justice system and the police inquiry.

Whatever this five-year police investigation may have generated – on this we cannot comment since we have not had access to the full documentation accumulated, on what was submitted by the RCMP to the Crown Law Office-Criminal (CLOC) – what we know is that there are reasons to believe that the CLOC did not feel completely at ease with the case as presented following the police inquiry. In December 2005, it requested the advice of an international expert (Dr. M.N.G. Dukes) as to whether there was enough documentation there to get an indictment. Dr. Dukes requested and obtained all the additional material, and provided an Advisory Report on February 12, 2006 (Dukes 2006).

On page 36 of this 41-page report, after an extensive review of the files, Dr. Dukes states unambiguously "I do not believe that there is in the documentary evidence available to me a sufficient basis for the criminal charges against Blood Transfusion Service [of the CRC] and its Director [Dr. Perrault]."

Despite this expert advice, the Crown still decided to bring the case to court. The Solicitor General brought to court one of four charges itemized by the CHS. In 2007, the case was heard by Justice Benotto and the parties indicted were exonerated on all counts in her judgment. This led to the other three charges being dropped by the Crown in January 2008, at the opening of the Hamilton trial meant to deal with them.

Again, it is difficult to believe that the doggedness and obstinateness in pursuing the indictment was not influenced by the broad movement of agitation and *pouvoir social* fueled by the CHS.

Does it amount to an indictment-seeking process?

It is difficult to witness this determination to indict (despite the expert advice suggesting that no condemnation is likely to be obtained) without recognizing what appears to be an undue sensitivity of the 'pre-justice system proper' to the pressure emerging from the CHS, the media and public opinion.

What we mean by pre-justice system proper is the whole process from the moment something untoward is noted or denounced, to the moment when it is brought in front of a judge. It goes from the fact finding by the police or other means (like commissions of inquiry), through the evaluation of the case by officials of the Crown in order to determine whether or not the matter should be brought to court. Ordinarily, one would expect the whole segment of fact finding to be conducted in complete independence, free from any interference by lobbies or other interested parties. In the same manner, the determination of whether or not the case should be brought to court should be made on the sole basis of the facts of the case, free of any direct or indirect interference or pressure from the outside.

Even though it may be difficult to prove direct interference in this case, it would certainly appear that there has been an impact of the *pouvoir social* on the decision to pugnaciously pursue the effort to indict these individuals, and to bring to court a case that was found to be groundless. Much of what we have brought forward in this book may be regarded as not full proof, but only a set of circumstantial evidence. But, as Henry David Thoreau would put it: "Some circumstantial evidence is very strong as when you find a trout in the milk."

References

Bang, Henrik P. 2003. *Governance as Social and Political Communication*. Manchester, UK: Manchester University Press.

Boudon, Raymond. 2005. *Tocqueville aujourd'hui*. Paris, FR: Odile Jacob.

Dukes, M.N.G. 2006. *Advisory Report*. February 12. 41p.

Ewald, François *et al.* 2001. *Le principe de précaution*. Paris, FR: Presses Universitaires de France.

Hubbard, Ruth and Gilles Paquet. 2007. *Gomery's Blinders and Canadian Federalism*. Ottawa, ON: The University of Ottawa Press.

Livermore, Daniel. 2010. "The Inquiry Model: Lessons from the O'Connor and Iacabucci Commissions," *www.optimumonline.ca*, 40(4): 1-28.

McDonald, Adam D. 2004. *Collaboration, Competition, and Coercion: Canadian Federalism and Blood System Governance*. A thesis for the M.A. Degree in Political Science at the University of Waterloo.

McDuff, Johanne. 1995. *Le sang qui tue*. Montreal, QC: Libre Expression.

Orsini, Michael. 2001. *Blood, Blame and Belonging: HIV, Hepatitis C, and the Emergence of Tainted Blood Activism in Canada, 1985-2000*. A thesis for the Ph.D. at Carleton University.

Orsini. Michael. 2002. "The Politics of Naming, Blaming, and Claiming: HIV, Hepatitis C and the Emergence of Blood Activism in Canada," *Canadian Journal of Political Science,* 35(3): 475-498.

Picard, André. 1995. *The Gift of Death.* Toronto, ON: Harper-Collins.

CHAPTER 4

| Modest General Propositions

I n this chapter, we suggest that the pathologies of governance discussed in the previous chapters might have been countered so as to avoid the tragedy, if a systemic perspective had been adopted. The fact that these repairs were not enacted then is regrettable, but it is hoped that they will be implemented should a new tragedy of this sort ever occur – and it will. Our optimism is based on the strong contention that, as Edward de Bono puts it, "once a new idea springs into existence, it cannot be unthought."

Fighting systemic governance failures

The amalgam of pathologies mentioned in the last chapter has revealed a fairly destructive dynamic of governance failure. It is not our intention to tightly partition the responsibility for the tainted-blood tragedy among those different factors mentioned in the last chapter, but it should be clear that we surmise that the bulk of the responsibility was borne by the 'venomous' factors. However, we do not ever wish to occlude the portion of the blame ascribable to the 'toxic' factors.

We suggest that the array of eight internal and external pathologies, explored above, have evolved through the unfolding of four broad perverse forces/mechanisms. Indeed, in our view, it is the compounding of these four forces/mechanisms that has produced the cascade that transformed the original crisis into a tragedy, the tragedy into a scandal, and the scandal into what might easily have been a major miscarriage of justice. Consequently, if our society is to be able to be better prepared for the next crisis of this sort, it must find ways to neutralize these four forces, and to find better mechanisms to handle them when our society goes through this sort of experience again – which is inevitable.

In the rest of this chapter, we identify these four sources of governance failure, show how central they have been in the blood tragedy, and suggest ways to neutralize some of these pathologies.

The unmet challenge of uncertainty governance[6]

The uncertainty that flows from the complexity of our modern world has blown away the simplistic analytical schemes of the past. We have mentioned, in chapter 1, some of the important pathologies of governance that it generated in the form of **the Forrester effect** (counterintuitive effects of action based on a poorly-understood socio-technical system), of **the Beck effect** (prevailing institutions responding adequately), and of **the Douglas effect** (the perverse view that every accident is caused by some person's criminal negligence). Recognizing this more enigmatic nature of our world, when it is plagued by deep complexity and deep uncertainty, has triggered a reframing of our way of dealing with governance: from a science of the precise to an approach to the imprecise (Paquet 2013a).

Deep complexity has impacted our world in three ways: **dynamically**, in the sense that problems can no longer be addressed piece by piece but as a whole; **socially**, in the sense that different perspectives and interests prevail, and actors must be engaged in resolving these issues and cannot ignore them; and **generatively**, in the sense that the future is undetermined, and old best practices are of no help – growing new practices is absolutely necessary (Kahane 2010: 5).

[6] This subsection draws freely from Gilles Paquet and Christopher Wilson's *Intelligent Governance – A Prototype for Social Coordination* (Ottawa, ON: Invenire 2016, chapter 1 (in press)).

Problem definition becomes more and more murky and results in its being ill-structured. Consequently it becomes more and more difficult to 'translate' such a messy situation into something that is analytically tractable. And when such a 'translation' is forcefully imposed on the issue, it most often generates a cartoon of a problem definition, one in which most of the substantively interesting and important features of the situation have been lost. In such cases, the manufactured version of the situation may appear to be analytically tractable, but the results are irrelevant or even toxic from a practical point of view, since the substantial aspects of the case have been lost in the effort to make the problem tractable.

One label has been used to capture the sort of problems generated in such circumstances of deep complexity and deep uncertainty – 'wicked problems'. The notion was first put forward by Rittel and Webber (1973), and has been used in various ways in the public administration literature since then (Paquet 1991). Roughly, it refers to problems where goals and objectives are ill-defined, and means-ends relationships are unclear and unstable.

Wicked problems evade clear definition. Rittel and Webber have defined them by a number of characteristics synthesized by Valerie Brown and further boiled down here, as follows:
- they have multiple interpretations from multiple interest groups;
- they involve trade-offs between multiple goals that are often ill-defined and unclear;
- they have no definitive solution;
- actions on this front lead to unforeseen consequences;
- the means-ends relationships in the actions taken are not stable;
- they are socially complex;
- they rarely sit conveniently within a discipline or organization;
- tackling them involves changes in personal and social behaviour;

- they cannot be generalized outside their particular context; and
- their formulation rests on paradoxes and calls for open inquiries (Brown *et al.* 2010: 62-63).

Recently, an approach better fit to deal with wicked problems has been adopted wholeheartedly by the Australian Public Service Commission (2007), and applied to the whole range of national policy decisions with great success. Indeed, it has been made the central feature of the analytical framework of Valerie Brown's research group at the Australian National University. The general strategy proposed by Valerie Brown (Brown *et al.* 2010: chapter 6) has the great merit of having served as a loose basic conceptual framework on which 15 short studies of wicked problems have been developed.

Each of the 15 studies starts with five questions:

- What is the wicked problem being addressed?
- What worldviews are involved?
- What ideals, facts, and ideas are contributed from the different types of knowledge?
- How have the diverse sources of evidence been brought together?
- What are the partial, uncertain, and open-ended findings from the study?

Valerie Brown's approach has proved useful in generating collective, open, imaginative, transdisciplinary inquiries. This is what will be required in the future when faced with the sort of problems that emerged with the tainted-blood crisis.

An equally powerful engine of analysis for wicked policy problems has been developed by the Centre on Governance of the University of Ottawa, and has been used to probe effectively a number of wicked problems (Paquet 2013b).

Whether one uses the Australian approach or the Canadian approach, the recently developed soft systems methodology offers promising avenues (Checkland and Scholes 1990). But it must be admitted that such approaches have not yet permeated the conventional ways in which such problems are tackled in Canada.

Pouvoir social and scapegoating

Developing a more sophisticated approach that embraces uncertainty will not deal with all the pathologies mentioned above. The variegated social environment often generates all sorts of information cascades. We mentioned earlier the forces unleashed by the *pouvoir social*, and the tsunami of opinions (not always sound and well-grounded) that are imposed on the public on the occasion of tragedies, and that are seemingly indomitable.

This sort of movement, fuelled by the media, often ends up in scapegoating initiatives, and, in the most chaotic circumstances, in kangaroo courts and hasty lynching expeditions. While we have not witnessed the most horrific forms of such cascades in Canada, the tainted-blood crisis has demonstrated this sort of momentum, and would appear to have left most of the actors completely stunned and unable to react in a manner that would have tempered this toxic movement. In fact, the usual *laissez-faire* that has accompanied such information cascades has had some important consequences for the political system, and echo effects on the justice system.

There is no easy way to interfere with this dynamic of civil society without running into totalitarian tactics that are obviously unacceptable in a democracy. However, it is equally unacceptable to allow rumours, malevolent gossip, and systematic and irresponsible disinformation to be disseminated by calumnious parties to contaminate the forum.

There used to be a time when one could count on a segment of the media to act as effective agents capable of and interested in disinfecting the debates, and clarifying the issues. One of the main lessons of the tainted-blood crisis has been that this countervailing power can no longer be counted on. In the issue of interest here, the media systematically fanned the flames, and certainly did not inject the sort of critical thinking one would have expected in the debates. The situation is likely to worsen in the future with the omnipresence of social media: one may foresee yet more toxic contagion with no self-controlling mechanism in sight. Consequently, ways will have to be found to avoid allowing organically emerging or manufactured, ill-founded information to dominate the scene and to disempower any rational discourse – obviously without extinguishing the freedom of expression and freedom of the media to disseminate what they think is appropriate.[7]

The irresponsibility and the unaccountability of the media have been denounced by Onora O'Neill and others. As O'Neill said, freedom of the press does not mean licence to deceive. The same can be said in their realm about lobbyists, politicians, intellectuals and ideologues. For the time being, those persons and institutions that are responsible for the dissemination of unfounded information or persiflage, and who hide behind the freedom of the press and freedom of discussion to deceive and disinform, are quite self-righteous, and there is no appetite for even the very meek criterion proposed by O'Neill (2003: 98) – assessable reasons for trusting and for mistrusting.

It is imperative that this question be addressed as a matter of priority if the forum is to be cleansed in the sense that Augeas' stables needed cleansing. It so happened that in the case of the tainted-blood tragedy, Justice Benotto was able to set the record straight. But it took years. Moreover, in the process, reputations were destroyed. Indeed, the choir leaders of the lynching party (who were the loudest voices calling in the front pages of the media for the punishment of the parties finally exonerated later) have often ensured that the content of the Benotto judgment, and the final outcome of this affair were reported on some back page of the same newspapers.

There used to be a time, 30 years ago, when we might have felt that competition among the media might suffice to ensure that the philosophy of 'fairly present' would prevail. Our experience in the recent decades, in the blood tragedy file but also in a large number of other files, has transformed our views. It would appear that nothing less than a true 'professionalization' of the

---

[7] The journalist who 'manufactured' the so-called $1 billion boondoggle at Human Resources Development Canada (HRDC) in Ottawa still writes his column, while many senior HRDC officials have been unwarrantedly and unceremoniously removed from their positions.

second oldest profession can make practitioners conscious of their burden of office, and refurbish journalistic standards to avoid the media becoming nothing more than whimsical agents of disinformation.[8]

The plight of monopoly and bureaucracy

A central source of the internal failures of the Canadian blood system at the time of the blood crisis has been the plight of monopoly and bureaucracy. We have shown earlier how the bureaucratic wrangles generated an extraordinary amount of waste and inefficiency. But another important source of difficulty has been the monopoly position of the CRC. In the United States, where a number of suppliers were competing in the blood market, there may have been, at times, reprehensible tactics, but there was also the constant pressure to offer to the customers a better product. This explains why, in many instances, the delays that were generated by bureaucrats and regulators in Canada did not materialize in the United States. Competition commands that the best quality product is supplied if a firm is to survive. Consequently, in the US, innovations were introduced as quickly as feasible, and improved products by one firm forced the other firms to adjust or face failure.

Some may say that we now have, in Canada, some form of competition between the blood system in Quebec and the one in place in the rest of Canada. We are sure that some emulation has emerged from it. But we are not certain that this has generated the optimal amount of competition as an agent of learning and innovation.

As for the bureaucracies, an effort has been made to respond to some of the criticisms put forward by the Krever Commission. While the new organizational set-up is perfectible, it may represent a form of organization that has been repaired 'at the meccano level' to ensure better control and accountability at the

---

[8] There has been a significant deterioration of the journalistic standards in good currency and a new hegemony of *doxa* over the duty of 'fairly present' in the recent past: one editor-in-chief of a Canadian daily could recently claim proudly and self-righteously that he had at critical moments abandoned in good conscience *l'impartialité* in the name of *la cause* (Paquet 2015).

operational level. However it is not clear that these repairs will suffice to eliminate all the blockages that may be said to have been responsible for the earlier catastrophe.

A blueprint for the redesign of the blood system was sketched in the fall of 1997 when Health Canada announced that it would manage the transition to a new system after the Krever report. A memorandum of understanding (MOU) was prepared in which the federal, provincial, and territorial governments recorded their guiding principles and accountabilities, and a transition bureau was created (with representatives from the provinces/regions, the federal government and a consumer representative). The MOU reconfirmed the seven principles adopted in 1989,[9] and added four new ones:

- safety must be paramount;
- an integrated approach is essential;
- accountabilities must be clear; and
- the system must be transparent.

It also established the National Blood Authority (NBA) – an incorporated entity with a board, empowered to borrow money. The NBA is responsible to the Canadian people, its members (as provincial and territorial ministers of health) to play a role similar to shareholders, and their responsibility is to do everything necessary to ensure access to a safe, secure, and affordable blood supply. The NBA was also provided with a mechanism to deal with emergencies.

---

[9] At the September 1989 meeting of the Interprovincial Conference of Ministers of Health, the CBC submitted its annual report which contained a refurbished set of seven principles meant to serve as the foundation for the Canadian blood system. These principles were couched in the form of 'wishes' rather than commitments that would have been truly binding: the voluntary donor system should be protected, national self-sufficiency should be encouraged, adequacy and security of supply should be encouraged, safety of all blood should be paramount, gratuity of all blood should be maintained, cost-efficiency and cost-effectiveness should be encouraged, and a national blood program should be maintained. This could not be interpreted as a mandated national blood policy.

The Canadian Blood Services (CBS) is a separate corporation, charged with the operations of the blood system. Its board is made up of contact persons from all the provinces and territories, and the CBS is dedicated only to the collection and distribution of blood and blood products. The ministers of health remain responsible for the use of the public funds they authorize, but they may *not* direct operational decisions. Moreover, the CBS was provided with considerable discretion to deal with crises.

On the bureaucratic front, the organizational redesign, following the Krever Commission, has only done some work to repair the structure of the blood system 'at the meccano level'. It has not been refurbished so as to immunize the system completely from the sort of rigidities at the interface between the policy and the operations levels, and between the diverse Treasury Boards and the financial needs ascertained by the NBA.

Commission of inquiry and the gate keepers to the justice system

The final zone of concern is the detectable promiscuity between the inquiry to establish the facts (by the police and other inquirers) and the decision, on the basis of those facts, to proceed or not proceed with the indictment, and the case being brought to court.

In the tainted-blood tragedy, there seems to have been some *confusion des genres*. Without in any way impugning the role of the police, the collection of facts was, at times, tainted, according to some of our interviewees, by a whiff of effort to find the basis for an indictment. In the same way, the constant presence of lobbyists in the corridors of the commission of inquiry might be regarded as unhealthy.

In both cases, even though there may have been nothing untoward and blamable reported, this may explain the somewhat asymmetric way in which prudence was used in choosing not only *not* to indict anyone (which is quite appropriate) but also *not* to exonerate on the basis of the material brought forth by the fact finding. In the case of the police results, an expert was asked to assess the proof by the Solicitor General, and it was found wanting. But this was not sufficient to persuade the Crown not to indict.

This leads to questions about the role of the gatekeeper who has to make a decision as to the next step. While it would appear that some prudence has been exercised by the Solicitor General's Office in the aftermath of the RCMP investigation (in asking for an external evaluation of the evidence), we remain uncertain as to whether the full extent of what had been revealed by the Krever Commission was brought to bear on the final decision of the Solicitor General, and to what extent the *pouvoir social* and the *zeitgeist* might have had an impact on the final decision to proceed to an indictment.

These speculative notes only point to the need to establish better safeguards to ensure total and complete separation among those different stages (from fact finding to indictment) to assure fairness to all parties, and to eliminate the possibility that public opinion and the whims of *pouvoir social* might ever again have an impact on the decision to indict. The problem is not academic. The Benotto judgment is only one of many cases in Ontario, where courts have thrown out indictments because it found them unwarranted. Given the immense collateral damages created by such 'mistakes' (indicting when there are no strong grounds to do so), it is crucial to ensure that they are minimized.

Lurking in the background is the possibility of culture governance having an undue impact: the possibility that an ideology based on the 'precautionary principle' might have found its way to contaminate the all-important decisions of the Solicitor General. As Justice Benotto says in her judgment: "... to assign blame where none exists is to compound the tragedy." This process is all the more objectionable when the trial gets unnecessarily dragged over months and months.

Brian Greenspan (the lawyer for Armour Pharmaceutical Co.) complained about the length of this 17-month trial – unnecessary prolix examinations, and the number of witnesses called by the Crown [the defence called no witnesses] –"a lot of them were superfluous, unnecessary and extended the trial well beyond what was reasonable."

David Scott (who defended Dr. Furesz) added: "When the public sees that criminal charges have been laid, it assumes that defendants are criminals. And when the court concludes that they are not criminals, the public says the justice system does not work. That's exactly what happened here."

The fact that Justice Benotto could say in her judgment that "The allegations of criminal conduct on the part of these men were not only unsupported by the evidence, they were disproved" could only lead some to conclude that "the trial was politically motivated" (Earl Levy, lawyer for Rodell) and might explain why some defenders have called for a public review (McPhee 2007).

*   *   *

All this shows that the repairs to the organizational and institutional apparatus in which the tainted-blood tragedy evolved are still far from complete. Some aspects of the 'meccano' of governance have been amended, but many other zones of concern remain murky. Consequently, it would be unwise to feel entirely reassured that another crisis of the tainted-blood variety would be handled satisfactorily. This remains a work in progress. Indeed, there is little hope that these repairs will be completed, unless the difficulties and pathologies raised earlier are approached with a systemic perspective ... and, on many of the fronts explored in this chapter, this would not appear to have been the case up to now.

Conclusion

Most certainly the Canadian blood system is better managed after the modifications that have been implemented as a result of the Krever inquiry. But it is not clear that it is 'governed' in a way that would immunize it from being lethally wounded by another unpredictable event of some consequence. This is because we still are not quite able to embrace deep uncertainty, nor have we developed an approach to policy that builds on it.

The same may be said about our inability to deal democratically with emotional and other unreasonable cascades that throw our democratic machinery out of whack.

Finally, we are also unable to approach realistically and critically our elaborate but quite imperfect machinery to handle the problems of responsibility and punishment in a deeply complex world, where there is not always one guilty party every time an unfortunate outcome materializes. From fact finding to indictment, too many things can go wrong.

In the tainted-blood tragedy, and in the case of other wicked problems, we seem to have a propensity to be satisfied with tweaking the management apparatus because it is the easiest thing to do. It may help, but one cannot get rid of the problem of governance failures by only tweaking the 'meccano'. As we have said earlier, a new approach is needed to deal with current wicked problems. Until the sort of revolution in the mind allows this new approach to be in good currency, we will remain saddled with governance failures with which we are not well equipped to deal.

References

Australian Public Service Commission. 2007. *Tackling Wicked Problems: A Public Policy Perspective*. Canberra, AU: Australian Government.

Brown, Valerie A. *et al.* (eds.). 2010. *Tackling Wicked Problems – Through the Transdisciplinary Imagination*. New York, NY: Routledge.

Checkland, Peter and Jim Scholes. 1990. *Soft Systems Methodology in Action*. New York, NY: Wiley.

Kahane, Adam. 2010. *Power and Love – A Theory and Practice of Social Change*. San Francisco, CA: Berrett-Koehler.

McPhee, Jennifer. 2007. "Public Review Called for in Tainted Blood Case," *Law Times News*, October 15.

O'Neill, Onora. 2003. *A Question of Trust.* Cambridge, UK: Cambridge University Press.

Paquet, Gilles. 1991. "Policy as Process: Tackling Wicked Problems" in T.J. Courchene *et al.* (eds.). *Essays on Canadian Economic Policy.* Kingston, ON: Queen's University School of Policy Studies, p. 171-186.

Paquet, Gilles. 2013a. "La gouvernance, science de l'imprécis," *Organisations & Territoires*, 21(3): 5-17.

Paquet, Gilles. 2013b. "Wicked Problems and Social Learning" in G. Paquet. *Tackling Wicked Policy Problems – Equality, Diversity, and Sustainability.* Ottawa, ON: Invenire Books, p. 59-92.

Gilles Paquet. 2015. "Failure to Confront," *www.optimumonline. ca*, 45(3): 16-32

Rittel, M. and M. Webber. 1973. "Dilemmas in General Theory of Planning," *Policy Sciences*, 4, p. 155-169.

CONCLUSION
| The Organizational Design Imperative

t is reasonable for the reader to feel less than fully reassured after reading Chapter 4. We have offered a plausible
and more reasonable reconstruction of the forces at work in
generating the tainted-blood tragedy than the fairy tale that
has been in good currency – courtesy of the lobbyists and the
media. But our response to the toxic and venomous forces
has fallen short of being fully satisfactory. We have provided
suggestions to counter some of these debilitating forces, but
for some others we may look as if we had little to offer – to
contain the malefits generated by crippling epistemologies
and *pouvoir social*, for instance.

Ergonomy will not suffice

The sources of the governance failures identified in the tainted-
blood affair were helpful in focusing on key dysfunctions at
work in our complex societies. But identifying broad zones of
concern cannot suffice. It is also necessary to propose reliable
diagnoses, and to proceed actively with the sort of particular
repair work likely to overcome the difficulties created by the
new generation of wicked policy problems confronted in
modern societies today. This is not necessarily easily done.

Some difficulties call for repairs of an 'ergonomic' sort –
like the latter two mentioned in the last chapter: bureaucracy
and monopoly, and the sort of mindfulness required to ensure

that no *confusion des genres* is allowed in the inquiry funnel that goes from problem definition and fact-finding to development evaluation, and the decision to indict persons or groups. While handling these challenges is in no way easy, one can readily conceive of affordances to "help people to think about, know and use something more easily and to make fewer errors" (Rao and Sutton 2008: 132). However, equipment redesign might not suffice to make the organization more resilient and *antifragile*.

Other difficulties call for repairs of a more 'fundamental' sort – like the first two mentioned in the last chapter (crippling epistemologies and *pouvoir social*) – for they reveal problems requiring not only some change in equipment, but a profound transformation in our way of thinking and in our way of behaving, if the difficulties are to be overcome. New cognitive tools and new forms of regulation are needed to prevent toxic *débordements* that can unduly limit the purview of the inquiries, or allow emotional cascades to swamp our organizations or social systems (Paquet 2009a; Boudon 2005).

These two types of difficulties pose quite different design challenges: micro-organizational tweaking in the first case, and macro-organizational reframing in the latter case. It has been possible to progress on the former front as a result of the trolley of investigations launched in the aftermath of the tainted-blood tragedy – they were mostly uncontroversial equipment modifications. On the other hand, little progress of consequence has been achieved on the latter front due to the fact that transformative reforms are always controversial since they entail not 'changes of degree' but 'changes of kind'.

If one is to gauge the effectiveness of social learning – not only by what has been learned from the tainted-blood tragedy experience in Canada, but also by what effective correctives to dysfunction and failure have been invented to ensure that the country will do better the next time, it is assaulted by an avalanche or crisis of the same magnitude – it must be clear that any reasonable observer has to be cautiously prudent in claiming success. Moreover, it should be clear that much more time will have to be spent learning how to redesign 'fundamentally' than to simply redesign 'ergonomically' in the future. Yet one has a strong sentiment that this is a lesson that has not yet been learned.

Only part of the repair job has been done

In no way can it be said that the full nature of the new difficulties generated by deep uncertainty in our more complex societies has been appreciated. We remain in denial *vis-à-vis* the new wickedness of the policy-making challenges, and of the need to improve our methods of inquiry to deal satisfactorily with the new learning needed. Moreover, there has been no sign that policymakers have progressed much beyond the old bow-arrow-marksmanship analyses of yesteryear. We are still a far cry from the bold experimentations that Australia has been willing to launch on this front.

Yet the cost of inaction is so high that some priority has to be given to demolishing the barriers blocking the road to the development of the new inquiring systems, and to developing improved methods of social learning that promise new experimentations.

On the first front, it is impossible to escape from the power of denial and the existence of mental prisons.

The reductive and mechanical method of diagnosing problems has led stakeholders to almost completely occlude the power of systemic self-organization, and the existence of outcomes completely disconnected from the intended objectives of any stakeholder. This blindness to the very existence of wicked problems entailed the prevalence of diagnoses inspired by ideology or crippling epistemologies, and a misguided tendency to ascribe unwarranted responsibility to persons or groups for all sorts of toxic outcomes for which they could not fairly be held accountable. That sort of scapegoating could only lead to the proposal of ineffective correctives.

On the second front, this has meant an ill-inspired loyalty to inadequate methods of dealing with wicked problems.

As we showed in presenting the case of the tainted-blood tragedy, any systemic analysis seeking to depersonalize responsibility for toxic outcomes has tended to be regarded by journalists and academics as a cop-out: not a fair and more sophisticated effort to analyze responsibility in complex circumstances, but as an illegitimate sleight of hand to avoid assigning blame to individuals that the uninformed but very agitated *magistrats de l'immédiat* (Lacouture 2005: 14) have already identified as their favourite candidates for indictment.

A plea for some intellectual refurbishment and for more gumption

The governance approach has developed over the years a new *manière de voir*, a particular analytical framework, a refurbished language of problem definition and resolution, a clinical apparatus to track the source of organizational dysfunction, and a mental toolbox to design adequate repairs. This has challenged the relevance of the traditional apparatus for policy analysis. It has also questioned the usefulness of simplistic notions like leadership and strategy, and proposed an alternative vocabulary, based on stewardship and design (Paquet 2009b; Martin 2014).

Governance embraces complexity and uncertainty instead of eluding them, and directly adopts a multidisciplinary and systemic perspective to deal with such problems. This is the approach that has been used in the case study of the tainted-blood strategy as a cascade of pathologies in this volume.

Yet, there has been a strong reluctance to accept this alternative governance approach in academic and media circles. This resistance has been the result of an unenlightened attachment to a cosmology of Big-G Government claiming that, in all sectors, someone is fully in charge (or should be), that this someone can be expected to have all the information, the resources and the power required to guide the organization in the direction prescribed by common values, and that this someone should be punished when failing in this task.

Our claim has been that no one had all the information, power and resources necessary to be fully in charge, and that the idea that the stakeholders had shared values is a myth. As a result, we have raised serious concern about the ascendency of the 'precautionary principle', for instance. When this principle was judiciarized and transformed into an *être de raison*, claiming to gauge what experts should be expected to know in the abstract, and should be held accountable for in reality, social sciences entered Kafkaland.

But, one might say, what can be done about issues for which there are no meaningful ergonomic responses, and for which nothing less than a revolution in the mind will do, a rekindling of critical thinking capable of sabotaging the harm done by mental prisons and *pouvoir social*? We deal with this challenge in the postface.

Coda

Effective organizational stewardship is at best a work in progress, and it can only emerge as the result of a symbiotic conversation among stakeholders capable of eliciting the best possible evolving outcomes (that do not necessarily correspond to what was desired by any of the participants).

It only remains for us to reiterate that our short case study of the tainted-blood tragedy has exposed the flaws of the conventional storytelling about it, and has presented a progress report on what has been done in order to better prepare for the next crisis – while underlining that these repairs remain unfinished business.

References

Boudon, Raymond. 2005. *Tocqueville aujourd'hui*. Paris, FR: Odile Jacob.

Lacouture, Jean. 2005. *Éloge du secret*. Bruxelles, BE: Éditions Labor.

Martin, Roger. 2014. "The Big Lie of Strategic Planning," *Harvard Business Review*, 97(1): 79-84.

Paquet, Gilles. 2009a. *Crippling Epistemologies and Governance Failures: A plea for experimentalism.* Ottawa, ON: The University of Ottawa Press.

Paquet, Gilles. 2009b. *Scheming Virtuously: The Road To Collaborative Governance.* Ottawa, ON: Invenire Books.

Rao, Huggy and Robert Sutton. 2008. "The ergonomics of innovation," *The McKinsey Quarterly,* September 17.

PART II

The Benotto Judgment, October 1, 2007

This copy of the judgment was obtained from Dr. Perrault's lawyer, Greenspan & Partners, on October 1, 2007 after Justice Benotto handed down her judgment. This document will not be used for commercial purposes.

COURT FILE NO.: P51/04
DATE: 20071001

ONTARIO

SUPERIOR COURT OF JUSTICE

B E T W E E N:　　　　　　　　　　　　)
　　　　　　　　　　　　　　　　　　)
HER MAJESTY THE QUEEN　　　　　　)　Michael Bernstein, Robert Gatrell, Peter
　　　　　　　　　　　　　　　　　　)　Napier, Stacey D. Young, Chris
　　　　　　　　　　　　　　　　　　)　Dwornikievicz, Elizabeth Pereira and Peter
　　　　　　　　　　　　　　　　　　)　Fraser for Her Majesty the Queen
　　　　　　　　　　　　　　　　　　)
　　　　　　　　　　　　　　　　　　)
- and -　　　　　　　　　　　　　　　)
　　　　　　　　　　　　　　　　　　)
　　　　　　　　　　　　　　　　　　)
ARMOUR PHARMACEUTICAL　　　　　)　Brian H. Greenspan and Sharon E. Lavine
COMPANY, MICHAEL RODELL, ROGER　)　for Armour Pharmaceutical Company
PERRAULT, DONALD WARK BOUCHER,　)　Earl Levy Q.C. and Robin McKechney for
and JOHN FURESZ　　　　　　　　　　)　Michael Rodell
　　　　　　　　　　　　　　　　　　)　Edward L. Greenspan, Q.C., Julianna
　　　　　　　　　　　　　　　　　　)　Greenspan and David N. Tice for Roger
　　　　　　　　　　　　　　　　　　)　Perrault
　　　　　　　　　　　　　　　　　　)　Michael J. Neville and William F. Murray
　　　　　　　　　　　　　　　　　　)　for Donald Wark Boucher
　　　　　　　　　　　　　　　　　　)　David W. Scott, Q.C., Peter K. Doody and
　　　　　　　　　　　　　　　　　　)　Isabella Mentina for John Furesz
　　　　　　　　　　　　　　　　　　)

BENOTTO J.

REASONS FOR JUDGMENT

Page: 2

TABLE OF CONTENTS

Page: 3

Page: 4

Introduction

[1]   The evidence in this trial sought to reconstruct the unfolding course of events of the mid-1980s relating to the processing of a blood coagulation product used to treat haemophilia. It was commercially known as HT Factorate.

[2]   Charges of criminal negligence and common nuisance were brought against the corporate manufacturer of the product, one of its senior officers, the Director of the Bureau of Biologics in Canada, the Chief of the Blood Products Division and the National Director of the Blood Products Services of the Canadian Red Cross. The corporation is also charged with failing to report a deficiency under the *Food and Drug Act.* These accused were involved in the manufacture, licensing, and distribution of HT Factorate.

[3]   The events considered here were part of a disaster that gained national and international attention. It was often labelled "tainted blood." It gave rise to civil law suits, an inquiry and much publicity. Strong emotions still abound.

[4]   But here, in the process of judging the conduct of these four men and one corporation, discipline is required to ensure that subsequently acquired knowledge is not imported into the analysis. Sir Winston Churchill, in other circumstances, said:

> It is not given to human beings... to foresee or to predict to any large extent the unfolding course of events. In one phase men seem to have been right, in another they seem to have been wrong. Then again, a few years later, when the perspective of time has lengthened, all stands in a different setting. There is a new proportion. There is another scale of values. History with its flickering lamp stumbles along the trail of the past, trying to reconstruct its scenes...[1]

[5]   So we embark upon the trail of the past, following the controversies, the developments and the knowledge in the medical and scientific world of over twenty years ago for this will establish the context in which the accused are to be judged.

Haemophilia

[6]   Haemophilia is a disease, primarily affecting males, where certain clotting factors called AHF[2] are absent from the blood. The most common clotting factors are factor VIII and factor IX. Factor VIII deficiency is called haemophilia A.

[7]   There was a time when haemophilia was fatal. A person with the disease would be unable to stop bleeding internally or externally. Often, he would bleed into joints causing severe crippling. Transfusions, initially life saving, would later lead to heart damage and early death. There was no effective treatment. His life expectancy was short.

---

[1] House of Commons, November 12, 1940
[2] Anti hemophilic factors

Page: 5

[8]   In the 1960s it was discovered that by freezing ("lyophilizing") plasma, factor VIII could be separated from other blood components.   A blood product known as cryoprecipitate was developed and used extensively to treat haemophiliacs.   Life was still difficult however. Everyday activities could cause a cut which could cause a bleed. The patient would regularly have to go to a hospital or clinic for infusions.

[9]   In the 1970s new biological concentrates were developed. Through a process known as fractionation, the constituent factors of plasma are separated and a clotting factor is produced. Whereas cryoprecipitate was derived from a single donor, concentrates were derived from the pooling of plasma from thousands of donors.

[10]   This was a huge change, described as a miracle for haemophiliacs.   It made possible home infusion instead of hospital-based treatment. The person could travel, have a normal life and a normal life expectancy.   Concentrates could also be used prophylactically to prevent bleeds. However, as would become evident later, the fact that concentrates were derived from many donors also increased the risk of transmission of blood-borne diseases.

Licensing Blood Products

[11]   In order to legally market a drug in Canada, the manufacturer must be licensed. In the case of a biological drug (such as factor VIII concentrates), the product must be licensed as well. The regulation of these biologics was governed by the Bureau of Biologics ("BoB"), a division of Health Canada. Dr. John Furesz was, during the 1980s, the Director of the BoB. Dr. Donald Wark Boucher became the Chief of the Blood Products Division in 1983. Dr. Boucher reported to Dr. Furesz.

[12]   Before a biological product can be licensed, the manufacturer is required to submit complete information on the safety and efficacy of the drug along with chemistry and manufacturing data to the BoB. This is contained in a new drug submission. Daryl Krepps was a screening officer at the BoB. She received and reviewed new drug submissions before forwarding them for scientific review and gave evidence at trial about this process. The Blood Products Division of Health Canada was the scientific review body with respect to new drug submissions. As part of the review process the Bureau of Biologics would independently test samples of the product to confirm consistency with the manufacturers' statements. If the information was satisfactory, Dr. Boucher would make a recommendation to Dr. Furesz. If acceptable, the manufacturer would receive a Notice of Compliance ("NOC"). Typically, there would be discussions between the Director (Dr. Furesz) and the Division Chief (Dr. Boucher) before a NOC was issued. It was not a unilateral decision on any one's part. Once the NOC was approved, it was forwarded to the Assistant Deputy Minister for signature and stamp.

[13]   Inspections of the manufacturing facilities were a condition of licensing. The authority to inspect was contained in the regulations to the *Food and Drug Act*. Generally, inspections were conducted yearly for facilities in Canada, biannually for those in the United States and every three years for those abroad.

Page: 6

The Canadian Red Cross ("CRC")

[14]   The Canadian Red Cross Society's Blood Transfusion Service ("CRC-BTS") was the distributor of blood products in Canada. In the 1980s it was comprised of 17 regional centers across Canada responsible for collecting and distributing blood products. Each regional center was led by a medical director. The medical directors were described as representing most of the knowledge and expertise in transfusion medicine in Canada. They reported to the National Director. The national head office was originally in Toronto but moved to Ottawa in 1987. The centers placed orders to the head office and distributed the products to hospitals, which in turn dispensed them to patients.

[15]   In the 1980s the BTS included the Blood Product Services, or fractionation department. It also included nursing, laboratory services, and the national reference laboratory. The Blood Products Services was responsible for the purchase and distribution of fractionated blood products including factor VIII concentrates. The CRC-BTS was advised by a medical advisory committee, comprised of a wide sampling of people involved in the blood system. This committee included physicians who treated haemophiliacs. Their role was to advise the National Director on the needs of the treating community and the needs of, and impact on, the patients.

[16]   Dr. Roger Perrault was the National Director of the CRC-BTS from 1974 to 1986. Essentially, he was in charge of the Blood Transfusion Service. In 1986 he became the Deputy Secretary General of Operations at the CRC. At the relevant time, Dr. Thomas Walker was the deputy director of Blood Products Services. He was joined by Stephen Vick in 1986. Both Mr. Vick and Dr. Walker testified. Others at the BTS were Craig Anhorn, a senior manager, Dr. Derek Naylor, a biochemist specializing in plasma proteins, Dr. Martin Davey, a clinical haematologist and serologist described as having impeccable knowledge of blood products and Dr. John Derrick, a specialist in protein chemistry and plasma proteins.

[17]   The Blood Products Services Department was responsible for maintaining supplies of plasma products and coagulation factors (including factor VIII). This included managing the accumulation and transport of Canadian plasma to fractionation plants in the United States and Canada, the return of products from those plants, and the eventual distribution throughout Canada to hospitals. The department was also responsible for negotiating contracts with commercial suppliers of blood products. Canadian plasma could only make up about 50 percent of the Canadian demand for factor VIII, leaving the remaining 50 percent to be purchased from other manufacturers as commercial product.

[18]   Barbara Dickson was responsible for the purchasing of fractionated products at the CRC BTS from 1983 to 1989. Her responsibilities included issuing tenders and purchase orders once a product was selected. Information would be provided to Ms. Dickson's department by the fractionation department, which would be assembled and issued to suppliers. This final document was known as a Request for Proposal or "RFP". Suppliers would respond with a tender that would be presented to the vendor selection committee.

Page: 7

[19]   Dr. Walker holds Ph.D. in biochemical engineering. He began working at the CRC-BTS in May of 1983 as the Deputy Director of Blood Products Services, reporting to Dr. Naylor. In 1985, he accepted the position of Director of Quality Assurance, and his responsibility was to ensure that all of the CRC's operations met regulatory requirements.

[20]   Mr. Vick began his career with the CRC-BTS at the Medical Center in Hamilton, Ontario in 1973 and worked for the CRC for 26 years. Mr. Vick was hired by Dr. Perrault as a full-time administrator at the center. He was then assigned to Dr. Perrault to manage the administrative set-up of a new center in Sudbury. Mr. Vick moved to the CRC-BTS National head office in Toronto in mid-1986 and became Deputy Director of the Blood Products Department. Upon the departure of Dr. Naylor in 1986, Mr. Vick became the acting director of blood products and reported to Dr. Davey. Mr. Vick's responsibility at head office was to ensure that adequate supplies of fractionated products were available for Canadian hospitals.

[21]   The Canadian Blood Committee was formed in 1981 to oversee and fund the Canadian Blood Programme. In 1983 the Secretariat to the Committee was formed. Dr. Denise Leclerc-Chevalier was the executive director.

Armour Pharmaceutical Company

[22]   Armour Pharmaceutical Company ("Armour") is an American drug manufacturing company with offices in Pennsylvania and Illinois. It manufactured HT Factorate, a factor VIII concentrate at its plant in Kankakee, Illinois, using plasma collected by Plasma Alliance. The plasma was collected from donors, who were paid for their donation, at licensed plasmapherisis centres. Plasmapheresis involves the removal of plasma from donors and the return of red blood cells and other blood components to the donor.

[23]   Plasma collected by Plasma Alliance was shipped to Knoxville, Tennessee and then on to Armour's manufacturing plant in Kankakee for pooling, concentration, manufacturing and labelling.   HT Factorate was licensed by the Bureau of Biologics at Health Canada and distributed in Canada exclusively by the Canadian Red Cross Society Blood Transfusion Service.

[24]   HT Factorate came in two levels of purity: intermediate purity which was called Generation I, and high purity which was called Generation II. Only Generation I was distributed in Canada.

[25]   Armour sold factor concentrate around the world: in the United States, Germany, Italy, the United Kingdom, Canada, Spain, Japan, France, Australia, Chile, Puerto Rico, Singapore and in countries in Scandinavia.

Page: 8

AIDS

[26] Almost everyone who lived through the early 1980s was acutely aware of the stigma, fear and misinformation that arrived along with the horrid disease which became known as AIDS.[3] As scientists were struggling to determine the cause of this ravaging illness, politicians were reducing their budgets and people were dying painful deaths.

[27] Unlike other infectious diseases, AIDS presented not with direct effects of the disease, but rather with secondary symptoms derived from a destroyed immune system. Typically those who contracted the disease would go through one horrible infection after another, be in hospital again and again, waste away and become so weak they could not get out of bed. In the early years, no one survived AIDS.

[28] There was and is no issue in this trial with respect to the bodily harm inflicted by AIDS.

[29] Today, with the advent of antiretroviral drugs, AIDS is no longer necessarily fatal. But during the long, arduous path to identifying the cause of AIDS so that treatment could be developed, many died.

Identifying the Cause of AIDS

[30] There are three major agencies in the United States that deal with diseases such as AIDS: the Centre for Disease Control (CDC); the National Institute of Health; and the Food and Drug Administration (FDA). They work well together, sharing information and research.

[31] The CDC is an arm of the United States government that deals with the issues of preventative medicine for the United States and around the world. It started exclusively with infectious disease outbreaks and then moved into the prevention of some chronic diseases. Its activities include surveillance and design of ways to prevent the disease from occurring. It employs epidemiologists, who are its backbone, to determine the extent, cause and methods of prevention of particular diseases. People all over the world look to the CDC for its expertise and the data it produces. It is a highly regarded agency charged with protecting the nation's health. It was referred to as the "gold standard."[4] Its scientists are recognized experts in their fields. Not surprisingly, the CDC became involved with AIDS very early on.

[32] The technology we live with today has made us accustomed to the instantaneous availability of information. It was not so in 1981. At that time, the CDC issued weekly reports called the Morbidity and Mortality Weekly Report ("MMWR") so that information could be quickly disseminated.

---

[3] It was not until the Washington meeting (referred to below) in July 1982 that the medical and scientific community agreed on the acronym AIDS for Acquired Immune Deficiency Syndrome. It is used here for simplicity and consistency.
[4] Anita Bessler: April 10, 2007, at 17045-17046

Page: 9

[33] The June 5, 1981, MMWR reported five cases of a very unusual and highly fatal disease in gay men. This was the first description of what would become known as AIDS. A task force was set up at the CDC.

[34] Dr. Donald Francis, a highly respected virologist joined the CDC in 1971. He had previously worked with cholera, Ebola, and small pox. He holds a Doctorate from Harvard University in microbiology/virology. In 1981 he was working in the hepatitis division of the CDC in Phoenix, Arizona. Dr. Francis was appointed to the AIDS task force. The following month, on July 3, 1981, the MMWR reported that Kaposi's sarcoma, hitherto a relatively benign cancer, was killing gay men in New York and California. Dr. Francis stopped the work he had been doing with respect to hepatitis. He began working on AIDS full time, within a few months had moved to Atlanta and has been working on AIDS ever since.

[35] On June 11, 1982 the MMWR reported that this new disease had spread to the heterosexual community and was doubling every six months. To Dr. Francis, it was like Ebola or cholera. It was a huge epidemic. They could not find the cause. To make matters worse, the United States had made budget cuts which affected his work. In these early days, research was terribly under funded. Dr. Francis testified about this period:

> For us at CDC, I would characterize it probably as hell. This was a huge epidemic ... someone, myself who had unfortunately or fortunately specialized in high mortality infectious agents, like plague and Ebola and the like, and cholera, this was one that ranked way up at the top and was one that was very frustrating in terms of finding the cause of it. As we got more and more laboratory work and from the political side of the United States, very unfortunate time to have a public health problem at a time when this was anti-government politics, and, therefore, getting the budgets necessary to deal with this disease was extremely hard. And so huge numbers of people like myself and others spend hours – early morning, late hours – working full-time on this, probably several hundred people at CDC at this time and the same in local health departments. Anyone who saw this disease knew it was bad and knew that it was terribly important to find the cause and to understand it fully.[5]

Dr. Francis testified that by June 1982, he and other members of the CDC task force believed that the infectious agent was being transmitted by blood and sex.

[36] On July 16, 1982 the MMWR reported that the disease was seen in haemophiliacs who had received factor VIII concentrates.[6] This also pointed to the infectious agent being blood borne.

[37] As of July 1982, there still was no universally used name to describe this new disease. Dr. Francis organized a meeting of the factor VIII and blood products component groups. It was held in Washington D.C. in July 1982. From that time on, the disease was referred to as AIDS.

---

[5] Dr. Francis: February 27, 2006 at 468, 469
[6] Exhibit 15

Page: 10

Those in the scientific community continued their search for the infectious agent of the disease. They were quite sure it was transmitted through sexual activity, bodily fluids, blood and blood products. They were also concerned about the haemophilia community. Dr. Francis told the participants at the conference that the consequences to the haemophilia population could be disastrous. There was no reliable test for the causative agent.

[38]   About ten days after the July 16, 1982 MMWR, a patient was admitted to hospital in Montreal. As chance would have it, he was the president of the World Federation of Haemophilia. He was admitted because he had high fever and suspected infection. Partly in response to this patient, Dr. Christopher Tsoukas, an immunologist at the Montreal General Hospital designed and organized a study to look at the immune system of people with haemophilia. His plan was to determine if the infection was acquired through blood products. At this point, there was no transmissible agent known so the study was directed to the immune system of people with haemophilia. One theory studied was whether people with haemophilia who had a lot of foreign proteins through the injection of factor VIII concentrates would have abnormalities.

[39]   The study began in the fall of 1982 with 32 patients who were all examined by Dr. Tsoukas. All of them were receiving lyophilized factor VIII concentrate. He concluded that the immune systems of otherwise healthy haemophiliacs with no symptoms were abnormal. Dr. Tsoukas also compared the immune systems of people that had received factor VIII concentrate with those who had received cryoprecipitate. The latter turned out to be closer to normal.

[40]   On December 10, 1982, the MMWR reported on two haemophiliac children who had contracted AIDS. To Dr. Francis, this meant that factor VIII concentrates could cause the infection. The same day another article also in the MMWR reported AIDS in a 20-month-old baby in California. The disease was contracted after blood transfusions which included donations from a healthy gay male who was subsequently found to have AIDS.

[41]   By the end of 1982, the doctors at the CDC believed (as earlier suspected) that the infection was in fact blood borne. Health Canada published an article in December 1982 recommending how to deal with AIDS patients. The recommendations were consistent with the disease being blood borne.

[42]   In the December 11, 1982 edition of the "Canadian Disease Weekly Report,"[7] Dr. Tsoukas reported on his study of the 32 asymptomatic haemophiliacs. His data showed that a substantial proportion of asymptomatic hemophiliacs show abnormal cellular immunity.

[43]   In January 1983 another meeting was held in Atlanta. The CDC was recommending donor screening of the established risk groups, including homosexuals and intravenous drug users. Dr. Francis wanted something to happen at the blood collection sites. He asked how many people had to die before action was taken. Dr. Tsoukas was there and presented his findings.

---

[7] Exhibit 1

Page: 11

[44]   Dr. Francis was frustrated that there were no universally accepted recommendations arising from the meeting. It was agreed that factor VIII was associated with transmission of the virus but Dr. Francis wanted the CDC to go farther. In a memo on January 6, 1983, he wrote that "post factor VIII receipt AIDS will occur in this country in the coming two years." He urged the CDC to make its own recommendations. He said that for haemophiliacs, "I fear it might be too late."[8] In the end, recommendations came out in MMWR and it was essentially agreed that factor VIII-associated virus was transmissible by blood products.

[45]   Meanwhile, on both sides of the Atlantic work, was ongoing toward isolating the virus so vaccines and therapeutic interventions could be developed. There was Dr. Francis working as head of the CDC–HIV lab; Dr. Robert Gallo at the National Institute of Health in the United States; Dr. Jay Levy at the University of California in San Francisco; and Dr. Luc Montaigner at the Pasteur Institute in France. Politics and competition among some of the labs made this a "very ugly" time[9]. Co-operation between the Americans and the French was strained.

[46]   In May 1984 Dr. Gallo published what came to be seen as a seminal article in *Science* magazine describing the causative agent of AIDS. The scientific community knew that a new retrovirus variously known as HIV or HTLV-III or HRI or LAV was linked with AIDS. From this point on, there was a general awareness that a retrovirus was most likely associated with this disease.

[47]   In July 1984 an oft-referred to article in *Science* magazine described the causative agent of AIDS and gave it the name HIV. [10]

Multi-Centered Study in Canada

[48]   The Laboratory Centre for Disease Control ("LCDC") in Ottawa is responsible for tracking epidemics. In 1984 it was heavily involved with AIDS research. Dr. Michael O'Shaughnessy of the LCDC had been to Dr. Gallo's laboratory at the National Cancer Institute in Bethesda Maryland. Through his colleague Dr. Peter Gill, he asked Dr. Tsoukas for serum samples taken from individuals who were at high risk for developing AIDS or those who did have AIDS. This was in order to test the new assays[11] that were being developed in Washington.

[49]   The World Federation of Haemophilia met in Rio de Janeiro in August 1984. Dr. Tsoukas spoke about the immune system of persons with haemophilia. He also presented data which showed that a high percentage of persons who had been treated with factor VIII developed antibodies to HIV. Dr. Tsoukas told the conference that over 90% of the patients that had received non-heat treated factor VIII had become antibody positive or had "seroconverted".[12] This came as a shock to those present. Dr. Tsoukas thought the reaction was a sign of denial.

[8] Exhibit 19
[9] Dr. Francis: February 28, 2006 at 624
[10] At various times the virus was called HIV, HTLV III, LAV and HRI. For ease of reference, I will only use the initials HIV.
[11] Method used to measure how much HIV is present.
[12] To "seroconvert" means to go from a negative to a positive status with respect to the antibody

Page: 12

[50]   In the fall of 1984, Dr. Tsoukas started a multi-centre study. The study was to determine what changes occurred in haemophiliacs with the use of blood products and to associate some of the changes with any infectious agents they would have come across, including HIV. The multi-centered study started in January 1985. Patients were added to the study over time. The results were eventually presented in May 1987.   What surprised Dr. Tsoukas was the shocking difference between those who used cryoprecipitate and those who used concentrates: 9% of the former were positive; 50% of the latter were positive. The percentage for the latter was higher if the concentrates from Canada were mixed with those from the United States. To Dr. Tsoukas it meant that there was a higher risk if the patient received American concentrates. At this point, however, he was only concerned with non heat-treated factor VIII concentrates.

Heat Treatment of Blood Products

[51]   By 1983, the major drug manufacturers were already heat-treating their products for hepatitis B. Armour treated its HT Factorate at 60°C for 30 hours. This temperature/time combination was known as 60/30.

[52]   All manufacturers were also working on methods of inactivating the AIDS virus. There was some controversy and concern that the heat activation would actually cause other problems, which would inhibit the effectiveness of the concentrate. Indeed, early on, the haemophilia community refused to consider heat-treating.

[53]   During 1984 and 1985 there was a great deal of research conducted to determine the effectiveness of heat treatment on the virus. As is customary in the scientific world, results are published to "get the word out."[13] It is important to understand what the state of knowledge was in the scientific and medical community during this time.

[54]   Dr. Bruce Evatt was the Director of the Division of Immunologic Oncologic and Haematologic Diseases at the CDC. In early 1984, he and Dr. Steven McDougal of the CDC began HIV viral inactivation experiments with factor concentrates. These studies were started by the CDC and then further experiments were conducted on commercial products from the drug companies called Cutter and Alpha.

[55]   The CDC did not know whether those products would be completely safe. The scientists assumed that the level of safety would increase and the risk of transmission would decrease with heat treatment, but by the end of 1984 they "had no idea."[14] They just knew that non-heat-treated factor VIII would be extremely dangerous for patients with haemophilia.   The preliminary results from the studies demonstrated that HIV had an extreme sensitivity to heat. The CDC wanted to get this message out. To do so, Dr. Evatt met with representatives of the National Haemophilia Foundation's Medical and Scientific Advisory Council ("MASAC"). The meeting was in early October 1984 and MASAC immediately recommended the use of heat-treated factor concentrates.

---

[13] Dr. Tsoukas: February 22, 2006 at 160
[14] Dr. Evatt: June 28, 2006 at 6641

Page: 13

[56]   On October 13, 1984 MASAC released a publication that suggested that HIV was sensitive to heat treatment and recommended that haemophiliacs switch to heat-treated concentrate. These recommendations were published in the MMWR. This was the first time that data was published on inactivation of HIV in factor concentrates. The publication confirmed that virally spiked samples of factor concentrate that had been lyophilized and heated at 60° C. contained no detectable virus after 24 hours of heating.

[57]   The message from Dr. Evatt and the CDC was heard loud and clear by the haemophilia treaters. By the spring of 1985 most haemophilia treaters had switched to heat-treated concentrates. This switch actually halted an epidemic. According to Dr. Evatt, "it stopped it cold."[15]

[58]   Dr. Evatt continued the studies. Representatives of Armour were most interested in his experiments. Dr. Fred Feldman from Armour had inquired about them. On November 29, 1984 Dr. Evatt wrote to Dr. Feldman. In that letter he described the process used in the experiment and outlined his preliminary results. The letter indicated that there was no detectable virus with a heat treatment at 60°C for 24 hours. Dr. Evatt's letter concluded:

> Because LAV appeared to be extremely heat labile, we believe that the procedures presently used by the manufacturers for heat treatment of hepatitis virus would adequately inactivate the LAV virus.

[59]   This letter was significant to Armour since its heat treatment of 60/30 exceeded the 60/24 process referred to in the studies. Dr. Evatt confirmed at trial that these results were the best available at the time.

[60]   In August 1985, Drs. Evatt, McDougal and others formally published the results of these studies in the prestigious *Journal of Clinical Investigation* ("JCP").[16] The article included the results of preliminary heat inactivation studies conducted by the CDC in the spring of 1984 and the collaborative heat inactivation studies conducted by the CDC, Cutter and Alpha later the same year. The authors concluded that the HIV virus appeared to be heat labile and that by heating factor concentrates, the transmission of the virus should be substantially reduced or eliminated.

[61]   The data contained in the article showed that there was a margin of safety in Armour's heat treatment process. It showed that HIV is inactivated at a rate of one log[17] every 32 minutes in lyophilized factor VIII when heated to 60° C. The results of the experiments on the commercial product showed that no detectable virus was found after heat treatment at 68°C for 24 hours and at 60°C for 20 hours. This led to the conclusion that there would be a 37-log reduction with 60/20 heat treatment. The article stated: "This should provide a large, if not absolute, margin of safety."

---

[15] Dr. Evatt: July 6, 2006 at 7337
[16] Exhibit 49
[17] A logarithmic measurement

Page: 14

[62]   To arrive at this conclusion, the authors extrapolated from the measured data, assuming a constant rate of inactivation. The Crown has argued that this was in error. Dr. Alfred Prince, who testified for the Crown, said that Dr. McDougal is a very fine scientist but "he goofed"[18] here. Dr. Prince said it was not justified to extrapolate because projections always "flatten out." The Crown alleges that in Dr. McDougal's article a year later, on August 11, 1986,[19] he agreed that he was in error. Actually, neither Dr. McDougal's article nor his testimony at trial supports this assertion. Dr. McDougal said that the factor IX product that was the subject of the second article, demonstrated a curved line of inactivation and it was difficult to extrapolate from a curve. He explained that if measured data is "not linear, it will not obey linear kinetics through extrapolated point forms".[20] He did not acknowledge an error.

[63]   In any event, even if the extrapolation was not justified, it does not follow that those who relied on it were at fault. The highly respected authors from one of the leading agencies in the world were discussing results in a relatively new and evolving area of science. This was the highest state of knowledge at the time. To attack their conclusions twenty years later is to wrongly apply hindsight. Even Dr. Prince did not make this critique at the time. Although Dr. Prince now claims to have come to a different conclusion, two months after the publication of the *JCI* article, he wrote: "it is difficult to explain the difference between the results reported by McDougal *et al* and (my) findings."[21] He did not say the results differed because Dr. McDougal wrongly extrapolated. I believe that Dr. Prince revised his opinion with the benefit of hindsight. He practically admitted this in cross-examination:

> I cannot tell you what I was thinking in regards to the linear extrapolation at that time. This is twenty years ago or more.[22]

[64]   Also, the reference to extrapolation was in the "discussion" part of the article. The raw data confirmed no detectible virus after heat treatment at 68/24 and 60/20, parameters that bracketed Armour's process.

[65]   Later that same year, on October 19, 1985, Drs. J. Petricciani of the FDA, Evatt and McDougal published a letter in *The Lancet* promoting the use of heat-treated product. The letter used existing data on the seropositivity rate of donors and the behaviour of HIV during fractionation and viral inactivation. An extrapolation was then made about the expected viral titre of a plasma pool and the required level of heat inactivation to obtain a safe product. Dr. Petricciani calculated how much virus may be in a pool, how much reduction was necessary and the amount of concentrate a patient is given. The authors calculated that the infectivity of a plasma pool would be five logs. They applied the CDC data and calculated that the minimum reduction of virus due to the lowest heat treatment method of 60/20 would be 20 logs. The studies were done with unscreened plasma (that is, it had not been tested for HIV). The authors concluded:

---

[18] Dr. Prince: September 20, 2006 at 8652
[19] *Exhibit 392*
[20] Dr. McDougal: October 10, 2006 at 9514
[21] Exhibit 368
[22] Dr. Prince: September 26, 2006 at 8941

Page: 15

There seems to be enough of a safety factor afforded by AHF heat treatment to permit the conclusion that LAV/HTLVIII is unlikely to be present in the currently licensed heat treated AHF, and that the use of such products should not result in additional cases of AIDS in persons with haemophilia.[23]

[66]   This article gave great comfort and confidence to Armour as it confirmed once again that its process of 60/30 was safe. As will be seen below, it also provided assurances to the regulators and distributors of blood products. The November 1984 letter of Dr. Evatt and the CDC data were used by Armour as part of its successful license applications around the world.

[67]   Nonetheless, the Crown contends that the defendants who relied on these articles were wanton and reckless. As with the earlier article, the Crown took issue with the CDC findings, alleging that the many assumptions made were erroneous and that Drs. Evatt and McDougal did not have direct knowledge of the processes used by the commercial manufacturers. The Crown argues that the data was not used in the US for licensing because the product was already licensed there and that the CDC does not establish industry standards. Once again, it was Dr. Prince who testified in support of the Crown's position.

[68]   It is suggested by the Crown that the calculations were done on the basis of limited data and that Dr. Evatt did not know about the unfavourable heat inactivation data obtained by Armour including the studies by Dr. Prince. I discuss in detail below my views of the studies of Dr. Prince and his evidence. As I conclude later, his studies were unreliable and I do not accept his evidence. The "second guessing" about the correctness of the CDC conclusions are inextricably wound up with hindsight. More importantly, all who had to make decisions about blood products cannot be faulted for relying on the CDC particularly as endorsed by the FDA. The article of October 19, 1985 was confirming that, based upon the state of knowledge at the time, all of the licensed manufacturers were using processes that bettered the results in the experiments. That was the belief of the CDC and the FDA.[24]

Dr. Levy's Studies

[69]   While the CDC studies were going on, Dr. Levy, another well-respected expert in HIV in San Francisco, was also doing experiments using mouse retrovirus as a model virus. He worked with Cutter which heat-treated the virus for this study. Dr. Levy published an article in *The Lancet* in September 1984 wherein he concluded that the retrovirus was able to withstand heat and that substantial inactivation was found only after samples of factor VIII had been heated for several hours at 68°C. Dr. Levy was surprised that the virus was so resistant to heat.

[70]   The Crown says this should have been a warning sign, especially to Armour. However, the article was effectively ignored by the scientific and haemophiliac communities as having no bearing on the sensitivity of human HIV. Dr. Levy then studied human HIV, again with Cutter's process. He wrote a letter to *The Lancet* that was published on June 22, 1985. He concluded that HIV was resistant to heat and that after treatment at 68°C for 30 hours the virus continued to

[23] Exhibit 46
[24] Dr. Evatt: June 29, 2006 at 7077

Page: 16

exist. It took, in his view, 48 hours of treatment at 68 degrees to reach a point where the HIV virus was not detectable.

[71]   On July 3, 1985, Christopher Bishop from Armour UK sent an interoffice memo to Dr. Michael Rodell and others attaching the June 22, 1985 letter from Dr. Levy. Mr. Bishop's letter said:

> It would appear from Table 2 of this article that a heat-treating process of 60°C for 30 hours would be ineffective in eliminating the ARV.[25]

[72]   Mr. Bishop testified that he was simply referring the matter on to the scientists as he was not qualified to assess the information from Dr. Levy. At Armour, it was viewed as a study done for Cutter, a competitor, and not a comment on Armour's product. Anita Bessler was Vice-President of Marketing for Armour and later Vice-President of Licensing and Acquisitions for Revlon Health Care which included Armour. She considered the Cutter study "marketing data."[26] It is not clear how much time Armour spent considering this information. The standard of review, however, is not perfection viewed with the benefit of 20/20 hindsight vision. There is no evidence that Dr. Levy's second study caused anyone in the medical, scientific or regulatory communities to question Armour's process or to reconsider the views of the CDC. Also, there was evidence to support Armour's process.

Armour's Tuckahoe Meeting

[73]   On October 15, 1985 Armour's Recombinant DNA Steering Committee met in Tuckahoe, New York. This committee's purpose was, in part, the development of factor VIII products. It was made up of employees and officers of Armour and an affiliated company, Meloy Laboratories. Dr. Rodell was present as were many of those who testified at trial. Most of the meeting was taken up with the topic of the heat treatment of Armour's product. Dr. Joseph Perpich, a lawyer and a physician, was the Vice-President of Planning and Development for Armour. He was the note taker at the meeting. He said there was a good deal of anxiety about the heat inactivation results and that detectible virus was found in the final heated product. The minutes of the meeting disclose that the changes in the heat treatment would cost millions of dollars. Dr. William Terry chaired the meeting. Dr. Terry was an immunologist from the National Cancer Institute. He joined Meloy Laboratories and was its President. Meloy did research and development for Armour.

[74]   By the time of this October 15, 1985 meeting, Armour had preliminary results from Dr. Prince. Dr. Terry is recorded as asking whether the FDA should be approached with the preliminary results from Dr. Prince. Dr. Rodell was recorded as saying it would be "unwise to go to the FDA without completing our own work first."[27]

---

[25] Exhibit 519
[26] Anita Bessler: April 10, 2007 at 17098
[27] Exhibit 483

Page: 17

[75]   The statement of Dr. Terry (who was not called as a witness) and the response of Dr. Rodell and ultimately Armour are relied on by the Crown in its allegation of wrongdoing.

[76]   The Crown alleges that Armour and Dr. Rodell knew at this point that their product was unsafe and chose to wait for more favourable results before informing consumers, treatment providers and regulatory bodies. To a large extent, the Crown relies on the studies and testimony of Dr. Prince.

[77]   Dr. Prince was an important witness for the Crown. The Crown alleged that his studies conducted in 1984 and 1985 showed that Armour's process was unsafe. Armour, instead of disclosing this or changing its process, is alleged to have buried the findings. In addition, as outlined above, his testimony at trial was relied upon to discredit Drs. Evatt, McDougal and Petricciani. It is therefore important to consider his testimony in some detail.

Dr. Prince: His Studies, His Testimony

[78]   The New York Blood Centre is a major voluntary blood donor center. It also fractionates plasma to make derivatives such as factor VIII. It distributes factor VIII to the haemophiliac community in New York area, a region which includes about 20-25 million people. It is the largest distributor in the U.S. after the American Red Cross.

[79]   Dr. Alfred Prince was, for 42 years from 1965 to 2006, the head of virology at the New York Blood Centre. During this time he worked on eliminating, inactivating and preventing the transmission of blood borne virus.

[80]   In 1983 he approached Dr. Gallo's lab to obtain HIV to experiment on viral inactivation. In the fall of 1984 he was asked by Armour to evaluate the efficacy of its 60/30 heat treatment of HT Factorate. Dr. Prince's approach was to get both Generation I and Generation II factorate from Armour in a freeze dried form, liquefy it, spike it with the virus, lyophilize it then send it back to Armour for heat treatment. It would then be returned to him to see what the viral kill was. A few weeks before Dr. Evatt's letter to Dr. Feldman, on November 19, 1984, Armour had retained Dr. Alfred Prince of the New York Blood Centre to conduct these studies. Armour hoped to establish that its 60/30 heat treatment process would kill 4-5 logs of virus. This was not including the inactivation that would result from the lyophilizing process.

[81]   Dr. Prince performed five studies. They were plagued with difficulties. After a longer than expected delay, he reported to Armour. The first report was in January 1985. He had evaluated both Generation I and Generation II samples. In both samples, the virus was not detected after lyophilization and heating. The virus stock used was unexpectedly low. The study was repeated. The second study was conducted in two parts: 2(a) dealt with Armour's factor VIII Generation II; 2(b) dealt with Armour's factor VIII Generation I. The first part was reported to Armour in April 1985. There, the amount of the HIV inactivation due to lyophilization alone was 0.5 log. Heat treatment at 60/30 inactivated an additional 1.5 logs leaving a total inactivation of 2 logs. The study showed that heating for 72 hours at the same temperature killed much more virus, more than one hundred times more than heating for 30 hours. The second part of the second study was also reported in April 1985, two days after the

Page: 18

first part. Dr. Prince concluded that the total inactivation of HIV in Generation I after lyophilization and heating was either 1.5 or 2.5 logs. Armour had expected a 5-log kill from heat alone.

[82]   Studies 3 and 4 did not produce measurable results.

[83]   Study 5 evaluated the effect of heating at 60 degrees in the dry state of infectivity of HIV in Armours Generation II AHF and Factor IX. The results revealed that HIV remained in Armour's product and that the heating alone was responsible for less than 1.0 logs of inactivation. When the heating was combined with lyophilization, the total effect was reduction of 3.7 to 3.9 logs.

[84]   The only experiment completed by Dr. Prince on Generation I was 2(b), the report of which was sent on April 5, 1985. At trial, Dr. Prince had great difficulty interpreting his results. There were several arithmetic errors which made his testimony confusing and difficult, if not impossible to follow. If it was difficult to follow at trial, with all the benefits of hindsight, I find it must have been equally difficult for Armour and Dr. Rodell to follow at the time.

[85]   Eventually, Dr. Prince concluded that the efficacy of dry heat by Armour was somewhat limited. He wanted to publish an article and sent his manuscript to Armour. It appears to have been received by Dr. Rodell on November 12, 1985. Dr. Prince said that Armour took the position he could not publish it because it violated their agreement. In fact, it was most likely not publishable since one of the hallmarks of valid scientific research is the ability to reproduce results. Dr. Prince was unable to adequately reproduce the results of his experiments.

[86]   Dr. Prince claimed to be annoyed with Armour and set out to repeat the experiments on behalf of the New York Blood Center using factor VIII manufactured there. Dr. Prince reported his findings with respect to this experiment in a letter to *The Lancet* published on May 31, 1986. In that letter he did not say the Armour product was unsafe, he did not provide data for the 60/30 method and did not mention any manufacturers. He did not call for any action, but suggested long term surveillance.

[87]   There is no evidence that the publication of this letter impacted the medical or scientific community. In fact, it appears not to have impacted Dr. Prince. His own organization, the New York Blood Centre continued to purchase and distribute Armour HT Factorate.

[88]   Dr. Prince testified that the Armour method had "relatively low effectiveness."[28] The Crown's alleges that Armour and Dr. Rodell had a duty to disclose this information from Dr. Prince. In my view, this was not what Dr. Prince communicated to Armour, or to anyone, for that matter. In actual fact:

- His letter of May 31, 1985 did not say that the Armour product was unsafe because he did not want to create fear in the haemophiliac community.

---

[28]Dr. Prince: September 20, 2006 at 8696

Page: 19

- He did not say that Armour was manufacturing an unsafe product. Instead, he said his *"private* feeling was this was not enough to make a safe product."[29] (Emphasis added)

- He had "no idea" whether or not the New York Blood Centre continued to buy Armour 60/30 factorate after his *Lancet* letter and did nothing to bring the matter to the attention of the purchasing department. He said that, as chief of virology, he had "no role in any decision making on distribution of factor VIII."[30]

[89] In short, the Crown would have Armour put more value on Dr. Prince's studies than Dr. Prince did himself.

[90] This was a time of great uncertainty. In the face of this, and in light of the clearly articulated studies of the CDC, supported by the FDA, it would have been unreasonable, if not irresponsible, for Armour to have thrust such confusing, incomplete and inconclusive information into the community.

[91] Dr. Prince's views articulated at trial were not only tainted by hindsight, they were substantially revised from his earlier views and opinions. In 1995, ten years after the experiments done for Armour, Dr. Prince issued a press release dated October 6, 1995. It was published in the Philadelphia Inquirer on October 23, 1995. It was a public statement with respect to the Armour studies. It said:

> Although some newspaper reports imply that Armour was negligent in continuing to distribute the original 60/30 treated product through 1987, I do not share this conclusion.[31]

[92] I believe that this is an accurate representation of Dr. Prince's views both in 1985 and 1995. His statement goes on to say:

> It must be remembered that our knowledge of HIV was very limited at the time. Actions taken then cannot be judged in light of our knowledge today.

[93] Inadvertently, Dr. Prince has summarized the position of the defence. If Dr. Prince felt Armour's product was not safe, he did not tell anyone. In cross-examination he was asked about the public statement and the following exchange took place:

> A. I think this statement, as I've said many times before, does not really reflect what I was thinking at all respects. This statement, I think, reflects a desire not to harm a given production facility, company. Uhm, but I think many other statements that I've made indicate that I was quite concerned that the product might not be safe when given in large amounts to large numbers of people.

---

[29] Dr. Prince: September 20, 2006 at 8697
[30] Dr. Prince: September 27, 2006 at 8959
[31] Dr. Prince: September 27, 2006 at 8973

Page: 20

Q. And you kept that to yourself; you kept that as your private thoughts and you permitted the New York Blood Center to distribute this as your public position and the position that you were prepared not only to distribute to the American public but to the scientific community as well? That's what you permitted the New York Blood Center to provide to the public; isn't that right?

A. Evidently.[32]

[94]   Dr. Prince produced studies that were unreliable, confusing and inconclusive. He could not possibly have thought that Armour's product was unsafe or he would not have allowed his own organization to continue to distribute it. Nor would he have clarified his position in a press release 10 years later.

[95]   Armour and Dr. Rodell had a reasonable response to Dr. Prince's studies. It would have been wrong for them to rely on or to disseminate those studies in any way.

[96]   For the reasons set out above, I find that Dr. Rodell's comments at the Tuckahoe meeting were reasonable. (I will come back to Dr. Terry's comments later.)

The Meloy and Ehrlich Studies

[97]   It was clear throughout the trial that studies and/or experiments had been done by Meloy Laboratories and by the Paul Ehrlich Institute. Regrettably, no one who had knowledge of either set of experiments was called as a witness.

[98]   Towards the end of 1985, Meloy Laboratories conducted heat inactivation studies for Armour. In monthly reports, Dr. Alain Schreiber provided updates as to the studies. The updates from 1985 to 1986 referred to the ineffectiveness of the 60/30 process and the benefits of a 68/72 process. No one was called from Meloy to explain the results of those studies. Thus, they are not before me. Dr. Terry of Meloy had certain comments attributed to him in the minutes of meetings.

[99]   Dr. Walker testified that the Paul Ehrlich Institute was a world-renowned research facility. He said: "in the area of virology, I would say that there are two recognized...authorities in the world: CDC in Atlanta and the Paul Ehrlich Institute in Germany."[33] There was peripheral evidence at trial indicating that the Paul Ehrlich Institute reported favourable findings about Armour's product. There was also peripheral evidence that Dr. Terry criticized those findings as well.

[100]   Dr. Terry was not called to testify. The Crown nonetheless sought to excise portions of his comments recorded at meetings to support its case. Those comments included:

---

[32] Dr. Prince: September 27, 2006 at 8973-8974
[33] Dr. Walker: May 24, 2007 at 18127

Page: 21

- His query at the Tuckahoe meeting as to whether the FDA should be notified about Dr. Prince's preliminary results; and

- His statement (referred to below) at the PEC[34] meeting in February about proceeding with the exchange of screened for unscreened product immediately.

[101]   The Crown does not mention the fact that Dr. Terry also criticized the Paul Ehrlich Institute results which were actually favourable to Armour. The Crown has made inferences from Dr. Terry's statements that support the allegation that Armour and Dr. Rodell did not discharge their duties. The Crown relies on Dr. Terry's statements as somewhat of a warning which was ignored. There is an equally plausible inference that can be drawn from his statements when considered in context.

[102]   In the dynamics of a meeting involving scientific data it would be expected, if not demanded, by responsible people that those present would be encouraged to express and discuss divergent views. One reasonable inference from Dr. Terry's recorded comments is that he played the role of "devil's advocate": always questioning, always testing. This is part of responsible decision making. However, decisions taken were done by consensus and it is obvious that Dr. Terry concurred in those decisions.

[103]   The Crown's position with respect to Dr. Terry's comments highlights the dangers of hearsay evidence, particularly taken out of the entire context.

[104]   Throughout the trial the Crown sought to have information about the Meloy Studies introduced indirectly. Reference was also made in submissions. It is ironic that the Crown would aggressively attack the findings of the CDC when those involved in the studies were called, yet assert that the Meloy studies could be introduced without explanation. The manner in which the Crown attacked the findings of Drs. Evatt, McDougal and others, underscored the need to have at least one participant in the study testify.

Request for Proposals by the Canadian Red Cross and the BoB Requirements

[105]   The CDC studies and related articles did not go unnoticed in Canada. On November 16, 1984, Drs. Boucher and Furesz on behalf of the BoB issued a telex to all fractionators indicating that all AHF products needed to be heat-treated. A month later, the BoB issued what has been referred to as a "position paper." It included the Cutter collaborative experiments with the CDC, confirmed that Cutter was the only company to have so far demonstrated that their product eliminated HIV and went on to assure the haemophiliac community that all manufacturers would be required to provide evidence that HIV was inactivated by their procedures. The paper said:

> ...we have informed the Canadian Red Cross that further reliance on AHF products that have not been heat-treated cannot be justified and that such products should be replaced with heat-treated AHF as soon as feasible...The Bureau is

---

[34] Plasma Executive Committee

Page: 22

requiring all other manufacturers to provide evidence that HTLV III is inactivated by their procedure.[35]

[106] The Crown sought to elevate this position paper into a requirement that data verified by the manufacturer be provided on its own product. The paper actually requires evidence of inactivation. The studies by Drs. Evatt and McDougal are such evidence. The BoB had received evidence establishing a 6 log kill for product following Armour's methods. The paper was meant to explain why the November 16 directive was made and was one of several presented at the conference.

[107] In late 1984, the CRC circulated a RFP to fractionators for the purchase of 40 million units of factor VIII. All manufacturers were required to submit heat inactivation data. The vendor selection committee of the CRC included people from the fractionation department, the national reference lab, the finance department and purchasing. Representatives of the CRC considered the manufacturers Cutter, Travenol, Alpha and Armour. They met with Armour on December 19, 1984. Memoranda of the meetings were prepared by Dr. Naylor. At both the Cutter and Armour meetings, scientists presented data on the inactivation procedures. Anita Bessler from Armour said that the company would not provide precise data as to its temperature and time parameters due to patent issues and patient confidentiality concerns. Instead, Dr. Feldman provided a general overview of the Armour process. Dr. Rodell and Armour then provided Dr. Feldman's chart documenting the CDC's collaborative studies with Cutter and Alpha. Dr. Walker assumed that the results applied to Armour's product.

[108] The vendor selection committee of the CRC decided to choose Cutter for 30 million units and Armour for 10 million units. Alpha and Travenol were rejected on the basis of price. It was decided to purchase from two suppliers to guarantee adequate supply as this was always a critical issue. Dr. Perrault approved the recommendation. Dr. Walker said that during the selection process, the meetings were open and everyone was able to voice an opinion. They always tried to reach a consensus. Once the committee decided, a recommendation was sent to Dr. Perrault who had "a keen eye for detail" and was not "just a rubber stamp."[36]

[109] On April 12, 1985 the BoB approved the package insert/monograph and issued a NOC for Armour HT Factorate. The product monograph for HT Factorate that had been submitted on October 30, 1984 by Armour contained the following words under the heading "Warning:"

> The possibility exists that Acquired Immune Deficiency Syndrome (AIDS), an immunologic disorder with extremely severe consequences, may be transmitted by blood, blood products, and blood derivatives including clotting factors. However, the causative agent has neither been identified nor isolated.[37]

[110] The Crown argued that this label was deficient and misleading because, by this time, U.S. scientists had announced the discovery of the virus thought to be the causative agent of

---

[35] Exhibit 151
[36] Dr. Walker: May 24, 2007 at 18271-2
[37] Exhibit 189

Page: 23

AIDS.[38] This, it is argued, was known to Drs. Furesz, Boucher and Perrault as well as Dr. Rodell and Armour when HT Factorate was licensed and distributed with this product label.

[111]   On November 27, 1985, the CRC sent out another RFP for the upcoming contract period and Armour submitted a proposal. This was the first RFP factor VIII concentrate that required that the plasma be screened for HIV antibody. The wording of the technical requirement for heat-treating changed from the previous RFP to now only include a process under conditions "acceptable to the Bureau of Biologics." Dr. Walker testified that the viral inactivity data was seen as "academic" because they did not intend to compare the processes but to accept the standards set by the BoB.[39] Armour was awarded a contract for 12 million units. An additional 12 million units was awarded to the American Red Cross.

[112]   On November 20, 1986, the CRC issued another RFP. This time, Armour was eliminated.

The Seroconversions

[113]   On May 1, 1985, Dr. Rodell advised the FDA that a donor from one of the Plasma Alliance locations had developed AIDS. This donor had contributed 20 times and his donations had been traced to 17 different batches of concentrate, some heat treated, some not. Armour planned, as a result, to withdraw all non-heat treated product, taking the view that there was no need to withdraw the heat-treated lots.

[114]   The American authorities were notified. Dr. Elaine Esber of the Office of Biologics Research and Review in the US agreed that there was no need to withdraw the heat-treated lots. Of the 17 contaminated lots, some had been distributed in Europe, including lots X57610 and Y60402.

UK Seroconversion

[115]   Dr. David Whitmore was a haematologist at the Lewisham Hospital and Director of the Haemophilia Unit. On May 10, 1985 he was advised by Armour that lot Y69402 had been distributed at Lewisham. On June 28, 1985 Dr. Whitmore wrote to Robert Christie, the Director of Clinical Sciences at Armour in the United Kingdom. He advised that one of his seven patients who had received the product had seroconverted. This patient had tested negative on January 17, 1985, received the product on February 5, 1985, and tested positive thereafter. Dr. Whitmore was not too concerned about the seroconversion at the time. He assumed that the virus was killed by the heat treatment and the positive test was the result of a reaction to dead virus. Dr. Whitmore testified at trial that the implicated lot of Armour was the cause of the patient's seroconversion.

---

[38] Dr. Gallo's article was published in May 1984; the article in Science magazine was in July 1984
[39] Dr. Walker: May 24, 2007 at 18162

Page: 24

Dutch Seroconversion

[116]   Dr. J.W. TenCate was the head of the Department of Haematology at the Academic Medical Center in Amsterdam. Dr. Cees Breederveld was another haematologist at the hospital who primarily treated children. In the spring of 1983, they commenced a study to determine if there was any difference in terms of safety between the use of paid and unpaid donor products and on the use of heat-treated products. There were 157 haemophiliacs in the study. All were HIV negative. Between 1983 and 1986, 20 patients seroconverted. All but one was related to the use of non heat-treated product. The remaining seroconversion was a haemophiliac who had received one of the contaminated Armour batches distributed in the Netherlands.

[117]   Drs. TenCate and Breederveld exchanged information with representatives of Armour. Dr. Breederveld withdrew the product from their hospital. On September 6, 1985, Dr. Rodell was informed by way of memorandum that Dr. TenCate's patient had seroconverted. Mr. Bishop from Armour U.K. was dispatched to speak to Dr. TenCate and to investigate. Mr. Bishop reported the results of his investigation to Dr. Rodell on October 30, 1985.

[118]   Dr. TenCate requested vials of the product to test on chimpanzees. Armour was not prepared to provide them without the approval of Meloy Laboratories. In any event, Armour believed their product safe because it had been tested and no virus had been isolated or cultured.

[119]   On April 5, 1986, *The Lancet* published a letter from Drs. TenCate, Breederveld and others about this seroconversion. The letter stated:

> Thus, seroconversion to anti-HTLV III positivity occurred in a patient using exclusively heat-treated intermediate and high purity FVIII concentrate of American origin. According to the manufacturers, one of the donors whose plasma was included in on of the transfused batches which was of intermediate purity, has developed AIDS. All other possible routes of infection were excluded.[40]

[120]   Dr. Evatt had a vague recollection of learning about this seroconversion in the Netherlands in 1986.

The Chapel Hill Seroconversion

[121]   Dr. Gilbert White was a haematologist specializing in blood coagulations in charge of the Haemophilia Treatment Center at the University of North Carolina at Chapel Hill.

[122]   In December 1985 he telephoned Armour and Dr. Evatt because he identified a patient thought to have seroconverted after receiving heat treated factorate product. The patient had been treated with cryoprecipitate in his youth but had not had plasma, cryoprecipitate or other blood factors since 1975. He was admitted to the hospital on June 30, 1985 and at that time tested

---

[40] Exhibit 335

Page: 25

negative. After this test, he received Armour HT Factorate. He tested negative again in late July. During a follow up at the haemophilia clinic in August, he tested positive.

[123]   Dr. Rodell investigated the heat treatment of the implicated lot and was in contact with the CDC. The lot had been made with a combination of screened and unscreened donations. Dr. Rodell also advised the FDA.

[124]   On March 15, 1986 *The* Lancet published a letter from Dr. White about this. He stated:

> ...the *possibility* remains that in this case, heat treatment failed to inactivate virus and immunity was in response to infectious virus...Another *possibility* is that inactive virus or viral fragments provoked the immune response. If viral material is present in concentrates, heat treatment might inactivate virus, but viral antigen might still be present in amounts sufficient to elicit an immune response. Seroconversion in this case would not signify exposure to active virus. Another *possibility* is passive transfer of HTLV-III antibody...Another final *possibility* is that the patient acquired HTLV-III through intravenous drug use...This case illustrates the need for further studies...(*Italics added*)[41]

[125]   Dr. White was exploring various possibilities. His letter highlights the immunization versus infection debate that was still an issue in March 1986. He does not suggest Armour's process was unsafe.

[126]   This particular patient did have other risk factors, primarily drug abuse. Dr. Evatt spoke to Dr. Rodell of Armour about this. Their discussion was typically direct and candid. They shared information. Dr. Evatt told Dr. Rodell that this patient was possibly involved in a fraud and that he may also have taken a blood product from Cutter, a competitor of Armour. Dr. Evatt said he had some problems with this case because there were other risk factors.

[127]   In the spring of 1986, Dr. Evatt then got a call, he thinks it may have been from Dr. Rodell, advising him of seroconversions in the United Kingdom also associated with the Armour heat treated factor. This was Dr. Whitmore's patient. However, there were other patients who took product from the same Armour lot who were seronegative.

[128]   All three seroconversions were investigated by the CDC. The CDC reported them to the FDA. All relevant information was disclosed to the National Haemophilia Foundation. Dr. Evatt had several discussions with Dr. Rodell. There was nothing kept secret.

[129]   The seroconversions were known to the CDC, The FDA, MASAC and the United Kingdom's Department of Health and Social Services ("DHSS"). Dr. Evatt testified that he consulted with Dr. Zuck of the FDA, Dr. Levine of MASAC and Dr. Rodell of Armour. Documents show he was also in contact with Dr. Peter Jones in the UK.

---

[41] Exhibit 334

Page: 26

The Newcastle AIDS Conference

[130]   Dr. Peter Jones was the Director of the Regional Haemophilia Comprehensive Care Centre for North of England in the mid-1980s. He had heard rumours of the seroconversions associated with heat-treated factor concentrates and organized an AIDS conference in Newcastle in February 1986. During the conference he voiced concerned about the possibility that heat-treated products were transmitting HIV. He did not name Armour publicly although he was concerned about its heat treatment. He had read Dr. Levy's publication, had spoken to other physicians and was aware of the seroconversions in the UK, Netherlands and Chapel Hill. As a result of his remarks, a number of organizations began their own investigations.

[131]   Shortly after the conference, Dr. Jones wrote to the DHSS Committee on Safety of Medicines about his concerns. This time he named Armour. Dr. Francis Rotblat was a haematologist and the senior medical officer responsible for reviewing pharmaceutical company submissions for DHSS. After receiving Dr. Jones letter, she contacted Mr. Christie at Armour. Mr. Christie promised to provide everything available.

[132]   Mr. Christie then went to see Dr. TenCate who admitted that it was possible the positive test was a response to dead virus. Mr. Christie also investigated the Lewisham seroconversion. He reported to Armour that the positive test might be the immune response to dead virus.

[133]   The Crown alleges that Drs Perrault, Furesz and Boucher were negligent in their conduct after the Newcastle conference. It is argued that they made no meaningful inquiries in early 1986. Had they done so, the Crown alleges they would have learned the following:

- Two patients who received HT Factorate batches containing donations from a known AIDS donor had seroconverted;

- One of the patients who received a contaminated lot was a patient in Lewisham who was HIV negative before receiving treatment, received two vials of the implicated lot, and had seroconverted approximately four months later. He had no other risk factors, and had not received any other products for a substantial amount of time before the last negative test;

- Dr Whitmore was the patient's treating physician and he believed that Armour HT Factorate Y69402, a contaminated lot, was the cause of the seroconversion;

- Another patient who received a contaminated lot was treated by Drs. TenCate and Breederveld. The patient had tested HTLV-III negative on numerous occasions previously, but had seroconverted by January 1985. The patient had received only Armour's HT Factorate for a year prior to that and had no other risk factors;

Page: 27

- Physicians treating this patient had contacted the company because they believed that Armour had caused the seroconversion and the product was unsafe;

- Upon learning of the seroconversion, the physicians requested that Armour remove the product from their hospital. Armour did so;

- Dr TenCate had requested vials of the implicated lot to inject into chimpanzees to see if an infection would result, but Armour refused to provide the material; and

- The last seroconversion occurred in a patient in Chapel Hill and was publicly reported by Dr White. The patient was hospitalized following a car accident. The patient was negative during his hospitalization, but tested positive a couple of months later. During his treatment he had received a substantial amount of HT Factorate. Although the patient admitted to past IV drug use, there were no clinical or physical signs of recent use. The medical staff at the hospital did not believe the patient was currently using drugs, or was in any other risk group. Dr White believed that Armour HT Factorate was the cause of the patient's seroconversion.

[134] These allegations ignore the facts that the Chapel Hill and Dutch seroconversions were reported in *The Lancet*. They ignore the fact that the medical community, including Dr. White, was unsure and calling for more investigation. They ignore the fact that Armour was fully open and cooperating with all the authorities, including the CDC and the FDA. Drs. Perrault, Furesz and Boucher did not have a duty to speak to every single person involved in the Newcastle Conference. As set out in more detail below, their investigations were careful and complete.

Armour's Internal Investigation: the PEC Meetings

[135] On February 20, 1986 the Plasma Executive Committee ("PEC") of Armour met at Fort Washington. Dr. Rodell and other executives of Armour and Meloy were there. The minutes of the meeting show that a review of the viral inactivation data was necessary because of doubts in the plasma community concerning the efficacy of heat treatment. Dr. Jone's comments at Newcastle were referred to.

[136] Dr. Terry presented the results of Meloy's HIV inactivation studies on Armour products and apparently told those present that "it appears that dry heat treating plasma may not be totally effective."[42] As a result, although the data was not absolutely conclusive, and comparisons of the methods were not yet completed, a decision was made to upgrade the heating cycle to 68 degrees for 72 hours. It was also decided that no product should be used if the plasma donors were not screened. The timing of the switch from unscreened to screened was discussed. The minutes of the meeting show that it was agreed to postpone the exchange:

---

[42] Exhibit 522

Page: 28

Since this may be an industry wide problem, pending BoB response, centers where unscreened product may have been delivered will not be contacted until the situation is clear.[43]

[137] These centres included Canada. It was also agreed that Dr. Rodell would review the Meloy data, which had been presented by Dr. Terry, with the FDA. Five days later, Dr. Rodell met with Dr. David Aronson of the FDA. The Meloy data and the seroconversions in UK, Amsterdam and Chapel Hill were discussed. Dr. Aronson stated that Armour's current heat treatment process was adequate relative to HIV and that the product need not be withdrawn from distribution.

[138] Two days after Dr. Rodell's meeting with Dr. Aronson, the PEC met again, on February 27, 1986. The purpose was to decide what action to take regarding the unscreened HT factorate, namely whether or not to withdraw it. In a four page memo reporting on the meeting, Dr. Rodell states:

> The consensus attained at that meeting was to initiate the following steps, in order to provide the haemophilia community with product reflecting as much added margin of safety as possible:
>
> 1.   The distribution of product derived from plasma not tested for Anti-HTLV III would be stopped, unless absolutely no adequate supplies of material produced from tested plasma were available.
>
> 2.   When adequate supplies of new product are in inventory, an exchange program will be undertaken. At that time, customers will be advised to exchange their existing supplies for product derived from tested plasma.[44]

[139] The Crown alleged[45] that the failure of Armour and Rodell to withdraw the product immediately represented a marked departure from the conduct of a reasonable person and of sufficient magnitude to give rise to a conviction of common nuisance. They were, it is argued, under a duty not to distribute unsafe product and at this point there was evidence that the product was unsafe.

[140] Since the exchange of screened for unscreened was made a few months later, in June, the Crown's submissions are that Armour should have immediately withdrawn the product in February 1986. The submission is based on Dr. Terry's comments as recorded in the minutes that unscreened product should not be used. Once again, the Crown seeks to excise Dr. Terry's statement in support of its position. He was not called as a witness. Others who were at those meetings were. It is clear that, at the end of the day, there was a consensus reached, which must

---

[43] Exhibit 522
[44] Exhibit 762
[45] This allegation was made for the first time in the Crown's written submissions.

Page: 29

have included Dr. Terry. His isolated comments in minutes, unexplained by him cannot amount to a basis to criticize the ultimate decision taken. (I refer as well to my comments about Dr. Terry above.)

[141]   It is clear from Armour's PEC meetings that Armour and its employees were acting in a responsible manner. Adequate supplies were necessary to effect the exchange. In fact, Armour was an industry leader in connections with the screening of blood products.

Follow up to Seroconversions

[142]   Armour UK initiated a follow up to the patients who had received product from lot Y69402. Mr. Christie reported that 12 patients had received this lot. Five of the 12 had been seropositive before receiving it and one died of unrelated causes. Of the remaining six only Dr. Whitmore's Lewisham patient had seroconverted. In addition that patient appeared to be physically healthy.

[143]   In early March, 1986, Dr. Rodell and others from Armour flew to the UK to meet with representatives of the DHSS including Dr. Rotblat. The purpose of the meeting was to discuss the safety of Armour's product. While the seroconversion of Dr. Whitmore's patient remained a concern, the DHSS was not completely certain it was caused by Armour's product.

[144]   Dr. Rotblat issued a report on March 4, 1986 which mentioned discussions with Dr. Ten Cate as well as the BoB in the United States. Based on this information, the DHSS came to the same conclusion as the FDA that no action on Armour products was necessary.

[145]   The Crown alleges that Armour did not provide all of the information to Dr. Rotblat, namely all the information about the Chapel Hill patient or the Prince conclusions. As outlined above, the FDA was aware of the Chapel Hill patient and that there were serious issues with the case. I have already explained why Armour was justified in not discussing Dr. Prince.

The Exchange

[146]   On June 23, 1986 Armour announced the exchange of screened for unscreened product. This is the exchange which had been agreed upon on February 27, 1986. Armour's Canadian agent distributed the information to the Bureau of Biologics and the Canadian Red Cross. Dr. Rodell's letter included the following statements:

> Armour Pharmaceutical Company has an ongoing policy to openly discuss issues associated with the care and treatment of the haemophiliac. One such issue is the potential for Anti-HTLV III seroconversion subsequent to administration of heat-treated clotting factor concentrates produced from units of plasma collected prior to implementation of Anti-HTLV-III testing.
>
> We have been made aware of three instances in which hemophiliacs have tested positive for Anti-HTLVIII subsequent to

Page: 30

the administration of H.T. FACTORATE ...however the circumstances surrounding each case prevent a definite conclusion regarding association of the use of the product with seroconversion.[46]

Dr. Rodell discusses the cases in UK, in Chapel Hill and in Amsterdam. He states:

> [with respect to Chapel Hill patient] ...received two units of packed red blood cells...questions have also been raised concerning the patient's personal history with regard to other risk factors...

> [with respect to the Amsterdam patient] ...reportedly received only H.T. FACTORATE....

> [with respect to the UK patient] ...the initial determination of seronegativity for Anti-HILV-III was made using unlicensed reagents and purported seropositive ELISA results using these unlicensed reagents.

Dr. Rodell then requests that product from unscreened plasma be exchanged for screened.

[147]   The National Haemophilia foundation (NHF) in the US was supportive of the exchange and endorsed the safety provided by heat treatment.

[148]   The Crown alleges that Dr. Rodell's letter was "skewed and selective" and did not accurately set out the known facts. In particular:

- The reference to "two units of packed red blood" in connection with the Chapel Hill patient was designed to suggest that this could be the cause of the seroconversion;

- The reference to "questions" about the patient's history was misleading as there was only one question, namely the possible IV drug use;

- In discussing Dr. TenCate's patient, he used the word "reportedly" before the information that he received HT Factorate;

- The wording with respect to Dr. Whitmore's patient refers to "unlicensed" reagents and "purported" seropositive results; and

- The letter omitted:

---

[46] Exhibit 508

Page: 31

o   the fact that both Dr. TenCate's and Dr. Whitmore's patients
     seroconverted after using HT Factorate made with plasma from a known
     AIDS donor;

o   the results of the Prince studies;

o   the results of the Meloy studies which indicated residual virus;

o   the decision to upgrade to 68/72;

o   the concern expressed at an Armour meeting in February 1986 that plasma
     from multiple hot (i.e. positive) donors could surpass the ability of dry
     heat treating to eliminate sufficient virus;

o   that he and others had been required to attend in the UK before the DHSS;
     and

o   that they were waiting to exchange until they had sufficient replacement
     product.

[149]   In addition, it is argued that the exchange was far too late in that it was eight months
after the Prince results, six months after the Chapel Hill information, nine months after the Dutch
notification and almost one year after notification of Dr. Whitmore's patient.

[150]   I do not agree that the letter was misleading. Armour was one of the first to make the
switch to screened product. The UK and Dutch seroconversions had been reported in the
literature. There was no need to include in house discussions that led to a corporate decision that
was reasonably and responsibly arrived at.

Canadian Response to the Exchange

[151]   The CRC received Dr. Rodell's letter and immediately called a meeting of the
recall/withdrawal committee. The withdrawal was carried out by Dr. Anhorn and staff in the
BTS centres. Dr. Walker monitored the progress. Once the plan was in place, Dr. Davey would
have informed Dr. Perrault since they worked as a team.

[152]   Dr. Davey circulated a memo to the medical directors of the CRC-BTC centres
explaining the withdrawal, and attaching the letter from Armour, a list of all the lot numbers
involved, an itemized inventory of each lot number issued to the centres and a draft letter to be
forwarded from the centers to the hospitals explaining the situation. Dr. Davey apparently felt
there was no need to withdraw the product. Dr. Walker agreed that the screening was an added
level of protection and that Armour was justified to rely on this distinction between screened and
unscreened product.

Page: 32

[153]   On July 22, 1986, Dr. Robert Card, the MASAC Chair in Canada wrote to Dr. Davey of the CRC about the withdrawal. In the memo he expressed concern that "the methods used in Armour factor VIII by implication might not be effective."[47]

[154]   Dr. Davey replied saying that Dr. Card had already received all the information available to the CRC and concluded: "the data I have seen suggest that their heat treatment is as effective as the other manufacturers for inactivation of retroviruses although the heating period is shorter".[48]

Donor Screening/Lookbacks

[155]   The Crown alleges that in the absence of an effective heat inactivation procedure or proof that heat treatment was killing sufficient virus, the defendants ought not to have relied on donor screening as a safety net to eliminate HIV from Armour's factor concentrates derived from pooled plasma. The time between infection and the detection of the antibody by laboratory tests is called the window period. Donor screening did not detect individuals with a high viral load when they were in the window period. This window period could last as long as six months. All of the defendants, it is argued, knew this. In addition, the tests during the 1980s were fallible and the defendants are alleged to have known this too.

[156]   Armour had developed a system of "lookbacks" to test donors who tested positive to see if they had previously donated. If so, the donations that had not yet been pooled were removed from the manufacturing process. The Plasma Alliance centres maintained records that enabled them to search back and trace prior donations of positive donors and send a lookback notice to Armour at Kankakee. The units would be identified and removed if they had not already gone into production. The Crown argues that many units thus identified were not in fact retrieved. Also, the Crown contends that Armour developed a self-serving policy of determining when a product was "in production" and thus not retrievable. Armour's policy was to retrieve only plasma units packed in shipping boxes. Once the units were removed from these boxes, they were considered in process.

[157]   Armour's lookback policy complied with FDA standards and was known to the FDA. The Crown's criticism regarding the designation of "in process" plasma is difficult to assess in the absence of any evidence as to the industry standards. There was no evidence about other manufacturers' plants, or from the FDA or the BoB in the United States. There was evidence about the "time sensitive" nature of the process and the need to move quickly or lose the coagulation effectiveness of the plasma. In any event, it seems as though the FDA was aware of this process. There is no evidence that the practice regarding the lookback deviated from the reasonable practices at the time.

---

[47] Exhibit 820
[48] Exhibit 820

Page: 33

The UK Withdrawal

[158]   During the summer of 1986, Dr. Rotblat became aware that the Chapel Hill case was associated with Armour HT Factorate. In September 1986 she was advised by Dr. Frank Hill of Birmingham Children's Hospital that two boys had seroconverted after receiving unscreened Armour product. She reported this to her superior, Dr. David Jeffreys. He was the Principal Medical Officer in charge of new drug licensing.

[159]   On October 1, 1986 Armour representatives were called to an emergency meeting in London. On October 3, 1986 Armour's UK representatives met with officials from the DHSS who were considering suspending the product if Armour did not voluntarily withdraw it. By this time, Dr. TenCate's patient had developed full-blown AIDS.

[160]   Two more meetings took place on October 6, 1986 when Dr. Rodell and others met in London with five members of the DHSS. Armour's data, presented at the meeting, indicated that the product was now donor-screened. They also advised that the new 68/72 heat treatment could be ready for the market in a few weeks.

[161]   Despite these assurances, the DHSS decided to require a withdrawal of the product and it was agreed that Armour would formally surrender their product licenses. Armour issued a press release announcing the withdrawal from the UK market. It included the following:

> On September 29th ARMOUR received a telephoned report that
> two haemophiliac patients in the U.K. had sero-converted.... Both
> patients had, for some months, been treated with Armour's heat-
> treated Factorate, which was manufactured from plasma collected
> before the general availability of...screening...[49]

[162]   Armour sent copies of this press release to Dr. Walker of the CRC and to the BoB on October 7. (Details of the response of the CRC and the BoB are set out below.)

[163]   The Crown alleges that Armour and Dr. Rodell should have provided the CRC and the BoB with more information including:

- that Armour was forced to withdraw its heat treated product to avoid having a license suspension;

- the DHSS knew of five cases of seroconversions, not just the two on Mr. Christie's memo;

- the medical director of Armour UK was concerned when told about the need for withdrawal and expressed no antagonism toward the DHSS;

- test results for 3 others patients of Dr. Hill's were imminent;

---

[49] Exhibit 710

Page: 34

- the Dutch patient now had full blown AIDS;

- the DHSS officials knew that the current product was screened and still wanted a withdrawal;

- other manufacturers had no reported seroconversions; and

- Armour offered to provide 68/72 to the UK.

[164]   On October 14, 1986, Mr.Christie went to the Birmingham Children's Hospital to investigate. His trip report included comprehensive details about the two patients involved. His report said that one of the two patients was probably product related, the other not. This memorandum was provided immediately to the regulatory authorities in Canada and the US.

[165]   By October 20, 1986, Dr. Rodell had been advised of a seroconversion of another of Dr. Hill's patients. It was a young boy with no other risk factors. The tests indicated that the seroconversion occurred by April 1986. Mr. Christie immediately advised the DHSS. Later, Dr. Hill advised of a forth patient who seroconverted. It is alleged that Dr. Rodell and Armour did not contact the BoB or the CRC with respect to these other seroconversions.

[166]   On January 13, 1987, the results of the HIV tests on two of Dr. Hill's patients were received by Mr. Christie and immediately disclosed to the DHSS.

[167]   Despite submissions to the contrary, I find that Armour's response was quick, concerned and professional throughout. The alleged omissions did not amount to matters that Armour had a duty to disclose. The events were happening quickly and Armour was responding appropriately and not hiding any information.

The Response in Canada to the UK Withdrawal

[168]   Dr. Walker received the press release about the UK withdrawal on October 7 or 8, 1986. He sent a copy to Dr. Perrault and others at the CRC. People immediately burst into action. The next two weeks involved a constant stream of conference calls, meetings and activity. The issue was treated as a priority. Employees at the CRC began to check inventory to determine if they had enough AHF products to fill demand in the event of a withdrawal in Canada. The actions at the CRC upon receipt of the press release were summarized by Dr. Walker as follows:

> From memory, it is very difficult to place events exactly -- place them exactly in time, ... 20 years ago. I recall that Dr. Davey, Mr. Vick and I held several meetings. We contacted -- Dr. Davey contacted colleagues from the U.K. We contacted the representatives of the Canadian Haemophilia Society or the Haemophilia Treaters Society. We contacted the BoB.... We tried to put together a full picture of what had led to Armour's action in the U.K., what it meant for Canadian patients, ... what the impact would be, both on, ... - in terms of direct safety and also on availability of product, mindful that non-availability of the product, of Factor VIII in particular, is itself a safety hazard, and we tried to, and

Page: 35

we worked with BoB to come to a consensus as to what action should be taken in Canada.[50]

The evidence of Dr. Walker, Mr. Vick and others confirms this response.

[169] The following day, Dr. Walker called Dr. Boucher to see if he had any information on the situation. Dr. Boucher did not. Dr. Boucher requested information from the CRC about existing inventory. Employees of the CRC went on a search for possible replacement product.

[170] At approximately 5:15 pm on October 8, 1986, Dr. Perrault learned for the first time about the UK withdrawal when he was briefed by Mr. Vick. Dr. Perrault instructed him to keep trying to find replacement product.

[171] On October 9, 1986 at 10:30 am Mr. Vick called Dr. Boucher to provide him with the requested information. Dr. Boucher requested more data from the CRC about the status of the Armour product received since April 1985. Dr. Boucher called Mr. McDade the President of Armour on October 9, 1986. According to the notes of the conversation, Mr. McDade said that Armour was developing a product which would be heated for a longer period. Dr. Boucher's notes of the conversation indicate that Mr. McDade did not have information as to when the patients seroconverted on the non-heated material.

[172] On October 9, 1986 at 2:30 pm, Mr. Vick spoke to Dr. Boucher and provided him with information that had been requested. Dr. Boucher indicated that Armour was in discussions with the FDA and they anticipated having a new heat-treated product licensed within a few weeks. At that point, it was suggested that Armour replace the product. Dr. Boucher apparently wanted to wait to speak to Dr. Furesz who was not available until the following day.

[173] The same day, Dr. Boucher called Dr. Leclerc-Chevalier at the Canadian Blood Committee to update her on the situation. He told her that there had been seroconversions in the UK but that the product had been heat treated, not screened.

[174] On October 10, 1986 at 9:45 am, Dr. Perrault met with Dr. Walker and Mr. Vick. Dr. Walker testified that Dr. Perrault was strongly in favour of a withdrawal of the Armour product. Later that morning, they participated in a conference call with Drs. Furesz and Boucher. Mr. Vick indicated that replacement product could be shipped by October 14 and they hoped the BoB could fast-track the approval process. Dr. Furesz wanted more information. He advised that the FDA was not going to withdraw the product because of concerns about the impact on the US market. Dr. Furesz indicated that the information from Britain was inconclusive because the transfusion history of the patients was unclear so it could not be tied directly to the Armour product. Dr. Perrault pressed the BoB for more information. Dr. Walker testified that the position put forward by Dr. Perrault was that there should be a withdrawal. The position put forward by Dr. Furesz was that such action could destabilize the world market and thus he opposed full withdrawal. Dr. Perrault requested this position in writing from Dr. Furesz. Dr.

---

[50] Dr. Walker: May 22, 2007 at 17892

Page: 36

Perrault gave instructions to Mr. Vick to buy 10 million units of the Cutter product in case the withdrawal went ahead.

[175]   Another conference call took place at 2:15 p.m.. Dr. Card of the Canadian Haemophilia Society was asked to participate.   Dr. Furesz indicated a concern of the FDA that a Canadian withdrawal would force the US to follow and a significant shortage would ensue. The FDA was going to meet in October 14, 1986, and it was decided to have another conference call after that meeting.

[176]   Dr. Rodell called Dr. Walker of the CRC on October 10, 1986. Dr. Walker was filling in that day for Dr. Perrault. He testified as follows:

> Dr. Rodell, indicated that Armour was aware -- ...that the Red Cross, ... was proposing to withdraw the Armour product from the Canadian market; that Armour considered that unnecessary and inappropriate; that if the Red Cross persisted, it would be seen as a defamatory action and would be -- and the company would take the appropriate legal action. I wrote a speedy memo recording that call, left a copy for Dr. Perrault to receive on his return, and filed the retention copy, and I'm not sure in which file. [51]

[177]   I pause here to note that Dr. Rodell's words to Dr. Walker were relied on by the Crown to suggest an aggressive stance or a lack of cooperation. This comment stands in isolation and complete contrast to all of the other evidence about Dr. Rodell's words and actions. The evidence discloses patience, and thoughtful, well-reasoned responses. The comment was four days after the withdrawal which resulted from what must have been a difficult meeting overseas. It is understandable that one intemperate remark was made at this pressure-packed time. It does not establish lack of cooperation or lack of concern.

[178]   On October 14, 1986 during yet another conference call, Dr. Walker spoke to Dr. Furesz who said he had received additional but inconclusive information from the UK according to which it appeared that the Armour product was all unscreened and that one patient may have received other product. Dr. Furesz spoke to Dr. Thomas in the UK who worked for the National Institute for Biological Standards and Control and received the information from him.

[179]   During all this time, the CRC was working on buying more replacement product. The efforts resulted in a sense that they had enough product to last for six months. Later in the day, Dr. Furesz indicated that he was now leaning towards a recall or withdrawal.

[180]   On October 15, 1986 Mr. McDade sent Dr. Boucher a copy of Mr. Christie's report about his visit to Dr. Hill and relating the details of the two boys who seroconverted. That information provided details about two patients: patient no. 1 was 11 years old, sexually immature and had no risk factors; patient no. 2 was 15 years old, believed sexually inactive. He

---

[51] Dr. Walker: May 22, 2007 at 17940

Page: 37

did have a history of treatment with cryoprecipitate. He received the non-screened Armour product.[52]

[181]   On October 16, 1986 after the FDA meeting, another conference call took place with Drs. Perrault, Davey, Walker, Furesz and Boucher and Mr. Vick. Dr. Furesz indicated that the FDA looked at the product's safety data and concluded it was adequate. The FDA was not going to require a withdrawal. In Dr. Furesz view, this fact, plus the inconclusive nature of the UK seroconversions meant that a withdrawal was not warranted. Mr. Vick recalled that Dr. Furesz had told him that the FDA undertook its own review of the viral inactivation data presented by Armour for its license and upon doing so concluded that it was safe. Also, Mr. Vick stated that Dr. Davey had been in contact with those involved in the UK cases and he was also of the view that a withdrawal was not necessary. Dr. Perrault supported a withdrawal until the very last meeting. Mr. Vick stated that, at the end of this meeting, Dr. Perrault passed him a note reminding him to ask for the BoB position in writing. In response, Dr. Furesz sent a written direction advising the CRC to re-issue the suspended Armour product. That letter reads:

> Following our review of the available scientific data, we concluded that the product, when prepared from plasma screened for HIV antibodies, is considered non-hazardous with respect to HIV infection in hemophilia patients. Consequently, we advise you to continue with the distribution of this product.[53]

[182]   On October 22, 1986, Dr. Davey on behalf of the CRC sent a memo to the Medical Directors at the Blood Services Centers in Canada advising of the BoB's position and indicating that the CRC would continue to distribute the current Armour product.

[183]   In response to concerns raised by members of the Haemophilia Society, Dr. Card who held positions with both the Haemophilia Society and the CRC responded to Bill Mindell of the Ontario Chapter of the Canadian Haemophilia Society. Dr. Card stated that the patients in question had received non heat-treated product from non-screened donors. The Crown argues that this statement was not reflective of the evidence to that date. Also, the Crown argues that the information received about Dr. Hill's patient the day before was not inconclusive and should have led to a withdrawal.

[184]   I find that the consultation and communication that was ongoing was extensive. The CRC was in constant discussion with the BoB which in turn was in consultation with the FDA. Also, there is also evidence that:

- Dr. Davey had consulted Dr. Forbes, the Chair of the UK Haemophilia Directors;

- Dr. Forbes had heard the presentation by Dr. Hill on October 9, 1986;

- Dr. Davey had contacted Dr. Bloom who knew the basis of the DHSS decision, who visited the FDA and who had spoken to the CDC;

---

[52] Exhibit 825
[53] Exhibit 805

Page: 38

- The FDA had the UK data; and

- Dr. Furesz had a close collaborative relationship with the FDA, with Drs Esber, Mayer, Parkman and Petricciani and they kept each other informed of scientific and regulatory matters.

[185]   The information about Armour was available to all regulators. The UK was the only jurisdiction to require a recall.

Armour's Move to 68/72

[186]   At the end of 1986, the manufacturing facility at Kankakee converted its heat treatment process from 60/30 to 68/72. Dr. Rodell indicated in the New Drug Submission[54] that all steps in the manufacturing process, with the exception of the heating of the final lyophilized finished product are the same as those provided for in the HT Factorate licence.

[187]   Dr. Rodell sent Dr. Boucher a copy of the application filed with the FDA to support the application to distribute 68/72. He included studies done by Meloy on both 68/72 and the previous 60/30. These results indicated less inactivation in the Generation I product and failed to reflect the 6-log kill Dr. Boucher had referenced in his original recommendation of HT Factorate in March 1985.

[188]   The Crown alleges that this information should have caused Dr. Furesz and Dr. Boucher to withdraw the product. Although licensed in the US, 68/72 was never licensed in Canada. Armour withdrew the application in favour of "Monoclate" another product that had been tendered several months earlier. This submission is therefore not relevant.

The BC/Alberta Seroconversions

[189]   In early to mid October, 1987, Dr. Walker and Mr. Vick learned of seroconversions in Western Canada. They immediately looked into the patient records and began withdrawing all products that the patients had received. On November 7, 1987, Dr. Walker wrote to the BoB announcing the withdrawal.

[190]   Both the CRC and the BoB worked together to share information, track down implicated lots and withdraw them. They were in daily contact. At the time, the seroconversions were not tied to one company and there was a concern about supply as the product was withdrawn.

[191]   In the fall of 1987, the BoB retained Dr. Robert Remis, an epidemiologist and public health specialist. Dr. Remis was told about the cluster of HIV infections among haemophiliac patients in British Columbia. He was asked to carry out an outbreak investigation or field investigation to determine the cause. In connection with this, he travelled to the Kankakee plant with Dr. Boucher. He learned that lots B71308, B71408 and B71508 had all come from the

---

[54] Exhibit 581

Page: 39

same donor. Dr. Remis testified that this was very important in arriving at an explanation. Soon after, on December 10, 1987 a formal recall of three lots of Armour HT Factorate was announced by the BoB. They were lots B71308, B71408 and B71508.

The Charges

[192]   Armour, Dr. Rodell, Dr. Perrault, Dr. Boucher and Dr. Furesz have been charged with four counts of criminal negligence, and one count of nuisance. Each count of criminal negligence is identical in its wording except for the time period covered (from 7 to 18 years) and the initials of the alleged victim. The nuisance charge covers a time span of over three years. The corporate defendant is also charged with a sixth count: that if failed to notify the Minister of a deficiency or alleged deficiency as required by the *Food and Drugs Act*.

Criminal Negligence

[193]   Counts numbered 1-4 have similar wording. The following is typical:

> Armour Pharmaceutical Company, Michael RODELL, Roger PERRAULT, Donald Wark BOUCHER, and John FURESZ, between October 1, 1984 and February 29, 1992, at the City of Toronto and elsewhere in the Province of Ontario, and in the Province of Alberta and elsewhere in Canada, and in the State of New York, and in the Commonwealth of Pennsylvania, and in the State of Illinois, and elsewhere in the United States of America, did, by criminal negligence, permit or cause to be distributed Armour H.T. Factorate infected with Human Immunodeficiency Virus (H.I.V.), which was infused into MM causing him bodily harm, contrary to Section 221 of the Criminal Code, R.S.C., 1985, c. C-46

The *Criminal Code* defines criminal negligence as follows:

> 219: (1) Everyone is criminal negligent who
>
> (a) in doing anything, or
>
> (b) in omitting to do anything that it is his duty to do,
>
> shows wanton or reckless disregard for the lives or safety of other persons.
>
> (2) For the purposes of this section, "duty" means a duty imposed by law.

Page: 40

[194]   The penalty for criminal negligence causing body harm is set out in section 221 which provides that:

> Everyone who by criminal negligence causes bodily harm to another person is guilty of an indictable offence and liable for imprisonment for a term not exceeding ten years.

[195]   Where criminal negligence arises from an omission, the defendant must be under a duty to do the omitted act. This is not the case where the criminal negligence involves the commission of an act.

[196]   The conduct of the accused must demonstrate wanton and reckless disregard for the lives or safety of others. This has been described as a marked and substantial departure from the standard of a reasonably prudent person in the circumstances. It involves an element of moral blameworthiness.[55]

"Wanton" has been described as:

- "heedlessly";[56]

- "ungoverned" and "undisciplined";[57]

- "unrestrained disregard for consequences";[58]

Reckless has been described as "heedless of consequences, headlong, irresponsible."[59]

Common Nuisance

[197]   Count 5 reads:

> Armour Pharmaceutical Company, Michael RODELL, Roger PERRAULT, Donald Wark BOUCHER, and John FURESZ, between October 1, 1984 and December 31, 1987 at the City of Toronto and elsewhere in the Province of Ontario, and in the Province British Columbia, and in the Province of Alberta, and in the Province of Manitoba, and elsewhere in Canada, and in the State of New York, and in the Commonwealth of Pennsylvania, and in the State of Illinois, and elsewhere in the United States of

---

[55] *Leblanc v. R.* (1975), 29 C.C.C. (2d) 97 (S.C.C.); R. v. J(.L.) (2006), 204 C.C.C. (3d) 324 (Ont. C.A.). *R. v. Waite,* [1989] 1 S.C.R. 1436

[56] *Regina v. Waite* (1996), 28 C.C.C. (3d) 326 (Ont. C.A.) at 341 per Cory J.A. (as he then was)

[57] *Regina v. Sharpe* (1984), 12 C.C.C. (3d) 428 (Ont. C.A.) at 430 per Morden J.A.

[58] *Regina v. Pinske* (1988), 6 M.V.R. (2d) 19 (B.C.C.A.) at 33 per Craig J.A. (affirmed on a different basis, [1989] 2 S.C.R. 979 at 979 per Lamer J. (as he then was)

[59] *Regina v. Sharpe*

Page: 41

America, did commit a common nuisance by distributing or failing
to take sufficient measures to prevent the distribution or infusion of
Armour H.T. Factorate, and did thereby endanger, through
exposure to the risk of Human Immunodeficiency Virus (H.I.V.)
infection, the lives, safety or health of the public, contrary to
Section 180 of the *Criminal Code*, R.S.C., 1985, c. C-46.

[198]   Common nuisance is defined, and the offence created, by s.180 of the *Criminal Code*. It
is as follows:

180(1) Everyone who commits a common nuisance and thereby

(a)   endangers the lives, safety or health of the public, or

(b)   causes physical injury to any person, is guilty of an
indictable offence and liable to imprisonment for a
term not exceeding two years.

(2)   For the purposes of this section, everyone commits a
common nuisance who does an unlawful act or fails to discharge a
legal duty and thereby

(a)   endangers the lives, safety, health, property or
comfort of the public; or

(b)   obstructs the public in the exercise or enjoyment of
any right that is common to all the subjects of her Majesty
in Canada.

[199]   Whereas the criminal negligence counts relate to specific individuals, the common
nuisance count relates to "endangerment" of the public. It does not require proof of actual injury
or damage[60]. The defence has acknowledged that if HIV was distributed to the public, it placed
the public at risk.[61]

[200]   While common nuisance may be satisfied by less egregious conduct than criminal
negligence, the offence still requires conduct that discloses a marked departure from an
objectively reasonable standard of care. The objective test was somewhat modified by Justice
Cory for the majority in *Regina v. Hundal*[62] to ensure that, "...the objective test should not be
applied in a vacuum but rather in the context of the events surrounding the incident". Justice
Cory elaborated by adopting the same standard as that of criminal negligence as described by
Justice McIntyre in *Regina v. Tutton*:[63]

[60] *R. v. Thornton* (1991), 82 CCC(3d) 530 (CA)
[61] Transcript May 7, 2007 at 17444
[62] (1993) 79 C.C.C. (3d) 97 (S.C.C.)
[63] (1989) 48 C.C.C. (3d) 129 (S.C.C.)

Page: 42

The application of an objective test...however, may not be made in a vacuum. Events occur within the framework of other events and actions and when deciding on the nature of the questioned conduct, surrounding circumstances must be considered. The decision must be made on a consideration of the facts existing at the time and in relation to the accused's perception of those facts. Since the test is objective, the accused's perception of the facts is not to be considered for the purpose of assessing malice or intention on the accused's part but only to form a basis for a conclusion as to whether or not the accused's conduct, in view of his perception of the facts, was reasonable...if an accused under s. 202 has an honest and reasonably held belief in the existence of certain facts, it may be a relevant consideration in assessing the reasonableness of his conduct...

[201]   The fault requirement for conduct in criminal law is mandated by the principles of fundamental justice as guaranteed by s.7 of the *Charter of Rights and Freedoms*.[64]

Count 6

[202]   Armour Pharmaceutical is charged alone with one additional offence. It is alleged pursuant to the particulars, that, under the direction and authority of Michael Rodell, it failed to notify the Minister of Health of a deficiency in its product. The indictment is:

ARMOUR PHARMACEUTICAL COMPANY further stands charged that between August 1, 1985 and December 15, 1987, at the City of Toronto and elsewhere in the Province of Ontario, and elsewhere in Canada, and in the State of New York, and in the Commonwealth of Pennsylvania, and in the State of Illinois, and elsewhere in the United States of America, failed to notify the Minister immediately of a deficiency or an alleged deficiency, in the viral inactivation process as described in the studies of Dr. Alfred Prince, concerning the safety of Amour [sic] H.T. Factorate, a licensed Schedule D drug manufactured by Armour Pharmaceutical Company and distributed to the Canadian Red Cross Society, as required by Section C.04.010 (b) of the *Food and Drug Regulations*, contrary to Section 26 of the *Food and Drugs Act*, R.S.C. 1970, c.F-27.

[203]   The Crown alleges that once Dr. Prince questioned the efficacy of the heat treatment process, the company was under an obligation to report this to the Minister.

---

[64] *(R. v. Naglik,* [1993] 3 S.C.R. 122 at para.36; *R. v. Hundal,* [1993] 1 S.C.R. 867 at paras. 42 and 43; *R. v. Gosset,* [1993] 3 S.C.R. 76 at paras. 31, 35-37)

Page: 43

The Victims

[204]   There is a publication ban with respect to the identities of the persons named in the indictment and others who received Armour product. The order is for the benefit of those persons, it is not meant to preclude them from self-identifying. Here, initials will be used.

The negligence victims

[205]   "MM" is named in count 1 of the indictment. He was born in December 1950 lived in Edmonton and seroconverted in 1987 at the age of 36. He died of AIDS related causes in 1992 at the age of 41.

[206]   His wife testified at trial and described the horrible course of his disease and the debilitating symptoms which caused him to develop blisters and sores and drop in weight from 150 to 90 -100 pounds.

[207]   While he was not part of Dr. Remis' initial investigation. Dr. Remis learned, in the course of his investigation about MM and believed that he had seroconverted as a result of the Armour product. In his opinion, the critical exposure period was from November 2, 1986 to October 13, 1987. During this period he received two types of factor concentrates, Cutter Factor IX and Armour concentrates from a paid donor. Dr. Remis was of the opinion that most likely explanation for his seroconversion was the product B71508 that he was infused with on January 30 and January 31, 1987. During his visit to the Armour plant in Kankakee on December 2, 1987, he learned that B71308, B71408 and B71508 were all made from the same pool. Since it appeared that 71308 and 71408 were contaminated, and given that they all came from the same pool, then B71508 was also likely contaminated.

[208]   "CL" is named in count 2 of the indictment. He was 15 years old when he seroconverted, having tested positive for the first time on September 22, 1987. He was not sexually active and not an intravenous drug user.

[209]   His sister and his father provided heart-wrenching testimony about the early stages of his life, his hemophilia, the development of AIDS and the resulting loss of his dreams.

[210]   CL was part of Dr. Tsoukas study. His medical records reveal that the exposure period for him was between December 9, 1986 and September 8, 1987. During this period he underwent a programme of immune tolerance induction which required large doses of factor VIII concentrates including 191 vials of Armour HT Factorate lot B71408. Based on his medical records, he likely became infected with HIV between December 9, 1986 and September 8, 1987. Within two weeks of the first dose of this lot he developed fever, a rash, fatigue and febrile illness. Dr. Remis testified that he was very certain that he was infected by the Armour lot. CL died in October 1995 at the age of 23.

[211]   "DH" is named in count 3 of the indictment. He was born in 1943. He tested positive for HIV in May 1983 but remained asymptomatic until 1987 when he became ill with a high

Page: 44

fever and flu-like symptoms. He was hospitalized in September 1994 and steadily declined in health until his death in February 1996 at the age of 43.

[212]   DH was part of Dr. Tsoukas' study. Unlike the other patients in British Columbia who seroconverted, he was an adult. He was married, denied any high-risk activity and did not use intravenous drugs. He received treatment for his haemophilia as an outpatient in the emergency room at Vancouver General Hospital. His first positive test was May 25, 1987, although it was thought that this was a mistake caused by a mix up of the samples. He developed an acute seroconversion illness on July 10, 1987 and it is argued that this is consistent with having seroconverted in June after the infusion of Armour lot B71408. Dr. Remis testified that he was very certain that DH was infected by Armour B71408 which he received in June 1987.

[213]   "JA" is named in count 4 of the indictment. He was born in 1974. He was 13 years old when he was infused with Armour product. He had no risk factors and had never received non-heat treated concentrates. He tested positive for the first time on July 21, 1987 at the age of 13. He received a diagnosis of HIV positive after using factor VIII products. Based on his medical charts, it appears he was infected between June 16, 1986 and July 7, 1987. During this period he received Cutter and Armour heat-treated concentrate. Within the Armour product he received lots B71308 and B71408. Dr. Remis testified that he was infected by one of the two Armour lots. He is the only named victim in the indictment who has not died.

[214]   JA testified by video link from British Columbia where he lives with his mother. He learned when he was a small child that he suffered from haemophilia. He initially had to go to the hospital to receive treatment with cryoprecipitate. Later, he was taught by Lois Lidner, the nurse at the haemophilia clinic in Vancouver, how to infuse concentrates at home. Currently he is at stage two of the AIDS progression and feels his health is pretty good.

The common nuisance victims

[215]   The Crown alleges that there were victims of the common nuisance in Ontario, British Columbia, Manitoba and Alberta. They were individuals who, in various ways were put at risk by the Armour product. With respect to the Ontario patients it is alleged that Armour distributed the unscreened product for six months after the decision to replace it. As such, the public was put at risk by Armour and Dr. Rodell. With respect to the B.C., Manitoba and Alberta patients, all parties agree that a long list of persons received Armour HT Factorate lot B71308, B71408 or B71508.

Causation

[216]   The Crown alleges that lots B71308, B71408 and B71508 were contaminated and that product from these lots caused the seroconversions of MM, CL, DH and JA.

[217]   Dr. Remis testified that his investigations in Kankakee and in Canada led him to this conclusion. In his analysis of the seroconversions in Canada, Dr. Remis created a "critical period of exposure" for each patient analyzed. That period was from three months before the last negative HIV test to two weeks before the first positive test. Dr. Milton Mozen gave expert

Page: 45

testimony that the latency period of the virus can be up to 27 months. If this is the case, then the infection period would date back to the non-heated era, prior to July 1, 1985. In addition, Dr. Remis acknowledged his previous statements that other drug manufacturers could be implicated in the seroconversions.

[218]   The Crown also relies on the evidence of Richard Pilon. After a long and scientifically complex *voir dire*, the results of the so-called "RNA" and phylogenetic testing were admitted into evidence. Mr. Pilon, under the direction of Dr. Sharon Cassol and at her lab conducted sequencing. Dr. Cassol designed the test but then relocated to South Africa, so did not actually take part in the hands on work.

[219]   The tests compared samples of the serum from Dr. Tsoukas' lab relating to patients who had seroconverted with vials of the implicated factor VIII lots. Both the serum and the vials were seized by the RCMP in 1999. The virus from these lots was sequenced and compared to the positive serum samples. Two samples from CL were sequenced. Mr. Pilon found that all of the serum samples were more closely related to each other than to any other HIV specimens and were likely derived from the same source virus. It is argued that this demonstrated that the HIV found in the Armour lots received by CL was in fact the HIV that infected him.

[220]   Additional testing performed by Mr. Pilon in 2004 in relation to another section of the HIV genome has confirmed these results. The samples (from CL and Armour) showed closely related sequences suggesting again that they originated from a common source.

[221]   The Crown argues that Mr. Pilon's evidence supports the study done by Dr. Remis and his conclusion that the infusions of lots B71308 and B71508 were responsible for the seroconversions of the patients.   It provides direct evidence with respect to CL and circumstantial evidence with respect to the others.

[222]   The Crown submits that there is overwhelming evidence of causation based on the following:

- Before receiving Armour HT Factorate, lots B71308, B71408 and/or B71508, each of the patients tested HIV negative;

- After using the implicated Armour lots, the patients tested HIV positive;

- Other than the use of blood products, the victims had no risk factors. Most were young and sexually inactive and there is no evidence of IV drug use;

- Lot B71308, B71408 and B71508 were made from the same plasma pool;

- Eleven donations entered Armour's plasma pool 713 during the six-month period before the donors who gave them began to test antibody-positive;

Page: 46

- There is a "window period" for HIV which precedes the emergence of detectable levels of antibodies. At this stage, the donor is highly viremic, but continues to test negative;

- Armour used the least rigorous heat-inactivation method;

- Lot B71308, B71408 and B71508 contained HIV;

- None of the tested products produced by Armour's competitors contained HIV;

- CL and DH experienced febrile illness consistent with acute seroconversion within two weeks of using the implicated lots; and

- The HIV from CL's serum is closely related to the HIV found in Armour's product.

[223] The Crown alleges that Armour HT Factorate caused the seroconversions which caused the bodily harm in the criminal negligence counts and put the public at risk in the nuisance count. I have a doubt about that assertion for the implicated lots were distributed elsewhere apparently without incident. I also have doubts about the efficacy of the phylogenetic testing. The samples were highly degraded. There were flaws in the study which rendered it inappropriate for forensic purposes.

[224] The issue is, however, academic. The law requires that the bodily harm or risk to the public be caused by the actions or inactions of the accused. There were no actions or inactions by the accused which showed wanton or reckless disregard for the lives and safety of others that in turn in caused the seroconversions. Likewise, there were no unlawful acts or failure to discharge legal duties which endangered the public. I have found that the conduct of the accused was reasonable throughout.

[225] If the imputed lots did cause the seroconversions (which I do not find as fact) then nothing that the accused did or did not do (within the meaning of the criminal negligence and common nuisance sections of the *Criminal Code*) caused those lots to be infected, licensed or distributed.

The Accused

Dr. Roger Perrault

[226] Dr. Perrault was the National Director of the Blood Transfusion Service of the Canadian Red Cross. The particulars alleged against Dr. Perrault with respect to counts 1-4 (negligence) are that he:

- Between November 21, 1986 and December 1, 1987 participated in the distribution of HT Factorate despite unfavourable laboratory results;

Page: 47

- Between November 21, 1986 and December 1, 1987 participated in the distribution of an inaccurate product insert;

- Between November 27, 1985 and December 1, 1987 failed to obtain information from Armour and from the BoB about Armour's processes; and

- Failed to inform others and failed to inquire into the safety of blood products being distributed.

[227]   The Crown relied on his job description to establish a duty to the public, a duty he allegedly breached. The job description includes:

- To ensure the highest possible medical and managerial standards are maintained in the operation of the BTS centres;

- To secure all accessible information to contribute standards, policies and long range plans; and

- To ensure that contracts with major suppliers meet quality and technical delivery requirements.

[228]   With respect to count 5 (nuisance), it is alleged that, between April 12, 1985 to December 17, 1987, he placed the public at risk of HIV infection by:

- Participating in the distribution of HT Factorate that potentially contained HIV;

- Failing to remedy the inaccurate label;

- Failing to obtain relevant information from Armour and the BoB; and

- Distributing unsafe blood products and failing to inform medical personnel and consumers about the safety of blood products.

[229]   The Crown alleges that Dr. Perrault's conduct showed a marked departure from the standard of care of the reasonable person and thus contributed to bodily harm and put the public at risk. The Crown alleges that Dr. Perrault was under a duty not to distribute unsafe blood products, to inform medical personnel and consumers of blood products about their safety and to inquire into the safety of blood products.

[230]   I reject the Crown's interpretation of the evidence and find, on the contrary, that the evidence taken as a whole establishes a thoughtful, careful and considered course of conduct by Dr. Perrault that has no element of blameworthiness.

[231]   Dr. Perault was considered a workaholic. His dedication to his work was often at the expense of his family and even his own health. He is an internationally respected scientist and an expert in transfusion medicine and science. He made decisions only after consultation with his

Page: 48

experienced top staff, in the context of a thorough analysis of the available information and only after careful deliberation. The medical information available at the time confirmed that screening plasma for HIV was an additional level of security. Dr. Davey was of the view that the Chapel Hill and Dutch seroconversions showed only a tenuous link to Armour and a withdrawal was unnecessary.

[232]   The Crown alleges that Dr. Perrault himself had doubts about screening, relying on statements he made that there were frailties in the screening tests. These comments on their own are equally consistent with a level of detailed analysis which questioned all the commonly held views. The evidence disclosed that screening issues were thoroughly studied by Dr. Perrault and the CRC and then implemented nation wide in September 1985. He would not have done this if he thought it was not to further enhance safety. This is an opinion that was widely held by the many experts who testified, including Drs. Tsoukas, Evatt, Jones and Breederveld. There is also evidence that the FDA held this view. As late as March 1987, it was reported in the MMWR that there were no reported factor concentrate-related seroconversions from donor screened plasma.

[233]   The Crown called no expert evidence on the standard of care. The Court is asked to infer that Canada should have followed the UK lead. However, Armour's screened Factorate continued to be distributed throughout the world. Moreover, the conduct of Dr. Perrault was careful and cautious throughout.

[234]   Intense consultation, careful consideration and a weighing of various factors related to public health marked the two-week period in October 1986 following the UK withdrawal. While Dr. Perrault was of the opinion that a withdrawal was necessary, he acted in consultation with the BoB whose scientists and administrators were considering the view of the FDA, the CDC and others on a worldwide basis. Dr. Perrault took the precautionary step of arranging for a contingency plan if a withdrawal or recall was ordered. Dr. Perrault instructed his staff to find alternative supplies in case of withdrawal. Only after the information from the FDA that the product was safe did he arrange to continue to distribute it.

[235]   There is no evidence that Dr. Perrault was under any duty to review labels, product inserts or monographs. This was the sole authority of the BoB. Even if he had been, my decision with respect to Dr. Furesz and Boucher below would apply to Dr. Perrault.

[236]   Dr. Perrault, through Dr. Davey, kept the hemophiliac community informed with respect to the relative risks of contracting HIV from HT Factorate. Dr. Davey followed the literature and kept the community advised of the events in 1986.

[237]   Far from establishing the requirements of either negligence or nuisance, the Crown has persuaded me that Dr. Perrault acted carefully and reasonably in regard to the health and safety of the hemophiliacs in Canada. He worked diligently in the interests of the hemophiliac community. He hired leading experts to work with him at the National Office and in the regional centres. He relied on the regulatory authorities and was in consultation with them on all the important decisions. They were forced to choose between distributing a product that was not risk free and leaving hemophiliacs without a life-saving treatment. Dr. Walker discussed the

Page: 49

balancing between risks and "non-availability of the product, factor VIII in particular is itself a safety hazard."[65] Although product had been obtained to replace Armour in the short term, it would have been irresponsible to de-stabilize the world market. A worldwide shortage would have been a potentially greater risk to Canada. Dr. Perrault analyzed, in painstaking detail, the various options, balanced the pros and cons and made a decision in conjunction with the regulators. He was put in a position of immense public trust. In that capacity he was thrust into a series of difficult events to which he responded with care, thoughtfulness and utmost professionalism.

[238]   The scientists at the CRC were confronted with a devastating disease which threatened to ravage the blood supply worldwide. It was a time of uncertainty with the medical and scientific knowledge constantly evolving. The causative agent of AIDS was discovered only a few years before many of the decisions herein were taken. By the time of the discovery, many hemophiliacs had already been infected.

[239]   Dr. Perrault's conduct has none of the elements that would lead to a finding of negligence or nuisance. Dr. Perrault acted properly and professionally throughout. The Crown has argued, somewhat ironically, that there was a foreseeable risk of harm. Of course there was. That is why Dr. Perrault took such care.

[240]   The Crown urges a cumulative look at the conduct of Dr. Perrault to establish a "continuum of liability." I have done so despite the defence submission that this is an inappropriate attempt to alter the standard of objective criminal liability. Having done so, I remain convinced that Dr. Perrault exercised care and diligence throughout such that would be expected from a person in a position of public trust.

[241]   Throughout the Crown's submissions, are lists of "meaningful inquiries" that Dr. Perrault failed to make. Had they been made, the Crown implies that the decisions made might have been different. While omissions can be the foundation for reckless conduct, it is unreasonable to suggest that Dr. Perrault and his staff had a duty to contact every single person who may have had information about the seroconversions. The scientists at the CRC were making inquiries on an ongoing basis throughout the time period in question. The hemophiliac community was represented by Dr. Card. Dr. Furesz consulted with his counterpart in the UK. Viewed in the context of what was and what was not done, Dr. Perrault's conduct was reasonable.

[242]   The Crown made improper references to the Krever Inquiry during submissions. Even if I took them into account, my decision would not be different.

[243]   Dr. Perrault is acquitted of all the charges against him.

---

[65] Dr. Walker: May 22, 1986 at 17892

Page: 50

Dr. John Furesz

[244]   Dr. Furesz was the Director of the Bureau of Biologics of the Department of Health of the Government of Canada.

[245]   The allegations against him, as particularized are as follows.

Counts 1-4 (criminal negligence):

(a) On or about October 30, 1984 to April 12, 1985, John Furesz and Wark Boucher, in Ottawa, Ontario, approved of the licensing of HT Factorate on the basis of inadequate documentation concerning the inactivation of HIV and the safety of Armour Pharmaceutical Company's manufacturing processes;

(b) On or about April 12, 1985 to December 1, 1987, John Furesz and Wark Boucher in Ottawa, Ontario, participated in the failure to withdraw HT Factorate's licensing in light of unfavourable laboratory results relating to HIV, HIV seroconversions associated with HT Factorate and the availability of alternative products, thereby allowing HT Factorate to be distributed in Alberta and British Columbia;

(c) On or about April 12, 1985 to December 1, 1987, John Furesz and Wark Boucher in Ottawa, Ontario, approved of the continued use of an inaccurate product insert/monograph respecting the safety of HT Factorate in relation to the risks posed by HIV and failed to remedy this with accurate information in a revised insert/monograph or other means of communication such as a label, communiqué, or press release;

(d) On or about April 12, 1985 to December 1, 1987, John Furesz and Wark Boucher in Ottawa, Ontario, failed to inspect Armour's manufacturing plant and to request of Armour and foreign regulatory agencies information concerning the inactivation of HIV and the safety of Armour Pharmaceutical Company's manufacturing process relevant to the withdrawal of HT Factorate and which could have been shared with medical personnel, haemophiliacs and their families in Alberta and British Columbia;

Duty for Omissions

(f) John Furesz and Wark Boucher had a duty to withhold or cancel licenses for unsafe blood products; to conduct adequate inquiries into the safety of blood products; impose conditions on

Page: 51

licenses to ensure safe blood products; and to enforce the regulatory scheme applicable to blood products.

Count 5 (nuisance):

(g) On or about April 12, 1985 to December 1, 1987, John Furesz and Wark Boucher put the public at risk of HIV infection by approving the licensing of HT Factorate on the basis of inadequate documentation concerning the inactivation of HIV and the safety of Armour Pharmaceutical Company's manufacturing process;

and by participating in the failure to withdraw HT Factorate's licensing in light of unfavourable laboratory results relating to HIV, HIV seroconversions associated with HT Factorate and the availability of alternative product allowing HT Factorate to be distributed in Ontario, Manitoba, Alberta and British Columbia;

and by approving the use the an inaccurate product insert/monograph respecting the safety of HT Factorate in relation to the risk posed by HIV and failing to remedy this with accurate information in a revised insert/monograph or other means of communication such as a label, communiqué, or press release;

and by failing to inspect Armour's manufacturing plant and to request of Armour and foreign regulatory agencies information concerning the inactivation of HIV and the safety of Armour Pharmaceutical Company's manufacturing process relevant to the withdrawal of HT Factorate or which could have been shared with medical personnel, haemophiliacs and their families in Ontario, Manitoba, Alberta and British Columbia;

Duty for Omissions

(h) John Furesz and Wark Boucher had a duty to withhold or cancel licenses for unsafe blood products; to conduct adequate inquiries into the safety of blood products; impose conditions on licenses to ensure safe blood products; and to enforce the regulatory scheme applicable to blood products pursuant to food and drug regulations, Part C, section 216, section 217 of the *Criminal Code*, *Public Service Employment Act*, section 23, Schedule III and the common law.

Licensing

[246] On March 26, 1985 Dr. Boucher wrote to Dr. Furesz:

Page: 52

The heat treatment procedure employed by Armour (60°C for 30 hours) differs from that of Hyland (60°C for 72 hours) and Cutter (68°C for 72 hours). The Armour heat treatment procedure has been shown to inactivate at least 6.0 logs of the human retrovirus, LAV. The procedure therefore meets the requirements for heat inactivation.

...

I see no objection to the issuance of a notice of compliance for this drug.[66]

[247]   This was a reasonable conclusion for Dr. Boucher, since it was based on the study done by the Centres for Disease Control. The state of the art of scientific opinion at the time was that the Armour heat-treating process was effective to kill the maximum amount of virus which was expected to be present in any plasma pool.

[248]   This represented the state of knowledge in the medical and scientific community at the time. Dr. Evatt testified that:

a)   His letter of November 29, 1984 to Dr. Feldman was widely disseminated because the CDC felt an obligation to get the information out as fast as possible because they wanted people to switch to heat treatment;

b)   The paragraph that included the words: "procedures presently used by manufacturers for heat treatment of hepatitis virus would adequately inactivate LAV virus" was put in the letter because the CDC believed it at the time;

c)   The results set out in the letter were the best available results at the time;

d)   The letter was the basis for the article in the *Journal of Clinical Investigation* in August 1985. That article included the following:

> Certainly, a procedure that reduces titre only 1 to 2 logs is insufficient to decontaminate Antihemophilic Factor because this reduction is obtained with lyophilization alone and lyophilized products transmit AIDS. However, the first-order kinetics of thermal decay and the long heating times, which are based on considerations for hepatitis virus inactivation (7) indicate an expected reduction of 37 logs at 60°C in 20 h (and even greater for higher temperatures and times). This should provide a large, if not absolute, margin of safety. [emphasis added]

---

[66] Exhibit 180

Page: 53

e)   in his article in *The Lancet*, of October 1985 it was confirmed that there was currently enough of a safety factor afforded by heat treatment in the currently licensed heat-treated AHF.

[249]   Dr. Tsoukas testified that he shared this opinion at the time. He also testified that it was generally understood that the FDA which licensed HT Factorate in the US on the basis of the CDC studies of Dr. Evatt and Dr. McDougal had high requirements and if they were met, it was an acknowledgment of achievement in terms of a product. The CDC was relied upon by agencies throughout the world. Dr. Levy's letter in *The Lancet* did not establish the state of scientific knowledge. In fact, it was largely ignored.

[250]   Dr. Furesz was perfectly justified in relying on the CDC information to license the drug.

Failure to Withdraw

[251]   The Crown alleges that HT Factorate should have been withdrawn from the Canadian market in 1986. The decision not to withdraw was taken after consultation with other regulators, with the CRC and its medical and scientific advisors, the FDA, and the haemophiliac community and its medical advisors both in Canada and elsewhere. His decision not to withdraw was one which was made by regulators around the world, except in the UK. He acted responsibly and reasonably throughout and there is no evidence of wanton or reckless conduct. While subsequent events may have shown that the decision could have been different, at the time, it was entirely reasonable.

[252]   In particular, Dr. Furesz had the following information:

•   The patient in Chapel Hill had a history of previous drug abuse and had been treated with various non heat treated product;

•   All three of the patients who seroconverted had been treated with unscreened product;

•   Even Dr. Prince's letter to *The Lancet* stated that his finding does not mean that dry heat treated products are unsafe with respect to AIDS transmission; and

•   The haemophilia community's advisors believed that screening was safer and provided an added level of security. This was supported by the clinical evidence at the time.

[253]   Dr. Furesz conduct in October 1986 after receiving the press release about the UK withdrawal was described in detail by Dr. Walker and Mr. Vick. That evidence discloses a careful, considered approach to a very difficult problem. Dr. Furesz was clearly balancing the potential risks of the product with the greater risks of a worldwide shortage. Dr. Walker best

Page: 54

described this analysis when he said that, although the position of the BoB was scientifically sound, some at the CRC had a "sixth sense" that it was the wrong decision. Eventually, however, the CRC came to the point of agreeing with the BoB. Dr. Walker said:

> The manufacturer said a recall is not necessary. The BoB said a recall is not necessary. We heard the FDA was not intending to do a withdrawal. We still felt there was a risk, but it would leave us in a position where we would have to replace the withdrawn product, and the purchase has a price. We would be spending Canadian health care dollars to address a feeling in the pits of our stomach.[67]

[254]   The Crown alleges that Dr. Furesz' concern about a worldwide shortage put the interests of US haemophiliacs before those in Canada, because at the time the replacement product obtained by the CRC was "safe and sound" in Canada. No expert evidence was lead with respect to regulation of drugs, yet the evidence discloses that the replacement product was for an interim period only Dr. Furesz was reasonably considering the long term affects of his decision. I infer that a worldwide shortage would ultimately impact Canada. This factor, however, was only one of many being considered by Dr. Furesz. He believed the product was safe. His belief was reasonable and shared by others.

[255]   Dr. Furesz had a difficult job to do, one that no one would have envied at the time. Whether he was right or wrong is not the point. The point is that he made a careful, reasoned analysis of the information available and did what his job required him to do: make a decision. That decision made on the basis of the facts before him was entirely reasonable.

Product Labelling

[256]   Dr. Furesz was advised by Dr. Boucher that the labels and product monograph for HT Factorate were satisfactory. They had FDA approval. They warned that patients might contract AIDS. They made no claim that the 60/30 method of heat-treating could totally eliminate the virus.

[257]   The labels accurately describe the significant risk of exposure to AIDS by using the product. There was no evidence that the label caused any patient to use the product who would not otherwise have done so.

Inspections

[258]   The Crown alleges that it was unreasonable for Dr. Furesz not to order inspections of the Armour manufacturing plant between April 12, 1985 and December 1 1987. There is no evidence to support this allegation. The inspections were not mandatory. Many inspections were not done due to cutbacks on funds and shortages of staff and a hiring freeze. Dr. Furesz could not hire his own staff or spend money or conduct inspections without authorization.

---

[67] Dr. Walker: May 24, 2007 at 18176

Page: 55

[259]   There was no evidence that any information uncovered during a routine inspection would have led to a different result. The visit to the Amour plant in December 1987 was an investigation specific to the seroconversions. It was not routine and did not mirror what would have occurred in a routine inspection.

Failure to Request Information

[260]   Dr. Furesz made extensive inquiries of Armour, the UK authorities, the FDA and medical and scientific advisors to the CRC and the haemophiliac community. There is no evidence that, had Dr. Furesz made more extensive inquiries, he would have obtained any more information that would have affected his decision.

[261]   Dr. Furesz is an internationally recognized scientist. He is a leading expert in fractionation. He is respected and has an excellent reputation for dedication to science and commitment to public health. He is held in high regard both personally and professionally. He called on all of those qualities during the difficult times surrounding these events. His conduct was thoughtful, careful and considered throughout. As such, his conduct did not fall within the meaning either charge of negligence or nuisance.

[262]   Dr. Furesz' counsel submitted that a criminal trial is an inappropriate forum to review the decisions of a public health regulator. Since I have found Dr. Furesz' conduct beyond reproach, I do not need to address this.

[263]   Dr. Furesz is acquitted of all the charges against him.

Dr. Donald Wark Boucher

[264]   The particulars set out above with respect to Dr. Furesz apply to Dr. Boucher. He was the Chief of the Blood Product Division of the Bureau of Biologics. He reported to Dr. Furesz.

Approval of HT Factorate

[265]   For the reasons set out above, with respect to Dr. Furesz, I conclude that Dr. Boucher's conduct in recommending the approval of HT Factorate was reasonable at the time. The Armour product was licensed around the world. There is no evidence to suggest that Dr. Boucher behaved differently from any other regulator in the world. There was thus no departure (marked or substantial) from the applicable standard of care. It is indeed ironic, as counsel point out, that the UK regulators, used by the Crown as a standard for the events of October 1986 licensed Armour's HT Factorate on the basis of the same studies and documents. Those studies and documents which I have extensively referred to represented the state of the scientific and medical knowledge at the time.

[266]   It was Dr. Boucher who requested that Armour's Canadian representative provide data from the studies. Olga Yacoub, who worked for Armour's Canadian representative, wrote to Dr.

Page: 56

Boucher. Her letter[68] both attaches Dr. Evatt's memorandum and copies his words exactly
stating:

> Based on these findings it appears the LAV is extremely heat
> labile; therefore our treating cycle of 60 degrees C for 30 hours
> developed initially against the hepatitis virus would adequately
> inactivate the LAV.

[267]   Although this data was said to be preliminary at the time of the correspondence, it was
published very shortly thereafter in the prestigious *Journal of Clinical Investigation*. Dr.
Boucher's personal stamp and initial appear on this document.

[268]   There is no basis to find that the conduct of Dr. Boucher in recommending a license for
HT Factorate was a marked or substantial departure from that of a reasonable person in the same
circumstances.

Failing to Withdraw

[269]   The information available to Dr. Furesz was also available to Dr. Boucher. For the same
reasons I find his conduct reasonable.

Labelling

[270]   For the reasons set out with respect to Dr. Furesz, I reject the Crown's position.

Failure to Inspect

[271]   For the reasons set out with respect to Dr. Furesz, I reject the Crown's position.

Failure to obtain Information

[272]   The Crown has not satisfied me that Dr. Boucher failed to obtain any information that
could be causally connected to the allegations in counts 1-5.

[273]   The Crown asserts that Dr. Boucher had a legal duty in relation to the safety of blood
products. In the opening statement, it was asserted that "he was to ensure the protection of the
Canadian public from health hazards arising form the use of these types of drugs."[69] This was
apparently a paraphrase of an unsigned job description for "Chief, Blood Products Division."
The Crown's position would require a public servant to virtually guarantee the safety of blood
products. This defies the evidence, which established that no biological drug can ever be
perfectly safe.

[274]   Dr. Boucher is acquitted of all the charges against him.

---

[68] Exhibit 442
[69] February 21, 2006 at 36

Page: 57

Armour Pharmaceutical Company and Dr. Michael Rodell

[275]   Armour and Dr. Rodell are also charged in counts 1-4 with criminal negligence for permitting or causing Armour HT Factorate infected with HIV and that was infused into four identified individuals causing each bodily harm.

[276]   Throughout the narrative of events numerous findings have been made with respect to Armour and Dr. Rodell directly in reference to the allegations against them. In each case, the allegations were rejected and there is a finding that they acted responsibly and reasonably.

[277]   The circumstances in the medical and scientific communities in the early 1980's were such that the conduct of Armour and Dr. Rodell was reasonable throughout. During the entire period of the particularized indictment, the following circumstances describe the context of Armour's manufacture and distribution of its 60/30 product:

- The medical and scientific literature supported the efficacy of viral inactivation through lyophilization and heat treatment utilized by all licensed manufacturers;

- The FDA, the primary regulator under whose scrutiny Armour's manufacturing facility and process was licensed, supported Armour's process and its responses to any concern raised;

- The accepted literature which affirmed that viral loads would not exceed five logs remained the standard against which the effectiveness of viral inactivation was measured;

- The dialogue between the haemophiliac community and Armour, particularly as represented by MASAC, evidenced the responsiveness of Armour and its complete compliance with all regulatory efforts;

- The disparate seroconversions associated with Armour were comprehensively investigated and reported to the appropriate regulatory agencies and led to action plans fully accepted and adopted by Armour;

- Plasma Alliance had been at the forefront of HIV testing so as to reduce even the theoretical possibility of significant viral loads;

- Action plans developed by regulatory agencies were fully accepted and adopted by Armour;

- Armour had initiated an exchange of all unscreened product for screened by the end of June 1986; and

Page: 58

- Counts 1 to 4 of the particularized indictment relate exclusively to fully screened product in relation to the three lots derived from a single pool of plasma.

[278] The particulars in relation to Armour and Dr. Rodell alleges as follows (emphasis added, in order to relate to the headings below):

1. That from July 16, 1986 to December 19, 1986 Armour, under the sole authority of Dr. Rodell, **used HIV infected plasma** received from Plasma Alliance in the manufacture of HT Factorate and failed to address the use of HIV infected plasma through particularized measures.

The significance of July 16, 1986 is that it marked the commencement of the collection of the blood donations by Plasma Alliance implicated in the Canadian seroconversions. The draw dates recorded on the laboratory reports indicate that these donations were received between July 16 and July 29, 1986. The significance of December 19, 1986 was that it was the date upon which the Canadian Red Cross received the third and final lot implicated in the Canadian seroconversions.

2. That from August 8, 1986 to September 3, 1986 Armour, again under the sole direction of Dr. Rodell, used **heat treatment** in the manufacturing of HT Factorate that was **of insufficient duration and temperature** to prevent HIV infection.

The commencement date of this particular, August 8, 1986, represents the date on which the plasma previously particularized was pooled at the Kankakee facility and received the designation Pool #713. September 3, 1986 represents the date that the manufacturing process for lots B71308, B71408 and B71508 derived from Pool #713 was completed.

3. That between September 3, 1986, (the date on which the manufacturing process for the three implicated lots was completed) and December 1, 1987, (the date on which Armour commenced the recall of all AHF treated by the 60/30 protocol) Armour, under the sole direction of Dr. Rodell, **distributed HIV** infected HT Factorate to its Canadian affiliates and to the Canadian Red Cross for distribution in Alberta and British Columbia.

4. That between the same dates, September 3, 1986 to December 1, 1987 Armour, under the sole direction of Dr. Rodell, **failed to withdraw** or recall its product in light of unfavourable inactivation studies and seroconversions associated with its product.

5. That between the completion of the manufacturing process on September 3, 1986 of the three implicated lots and the recall of 60/30 which commenced on December 1, 1987, Armour, under the sole authority of Dr. Rodell, used an

Page: 59

inaccurate product **insert/monograph** respecting the risk posed by HIV and failed to provide accurate information.

6. That between the date of the manufacture of the three implicated lots and the withdrawal of 60/30 Armour, under the sole direction of Dr. Rodell, **failed to notify** the Bureau of Biologics, the Canadian Red Cross, medical personnel, haemophiliacs and their families in Alberta and British Columbia of the risk of HIV infection posed by HT Factorate. The Crown further particularized that this alleged misconduct occurred while Armour and Dr. Rodell were under a duty not to distribute unsafe blood products and a duty to inform the various stakeholders with respect to the safety of HT Factorate.

Used HIV infected plasma

[279] The plasma received from Plasma Alliance on July 16, 1986 and thereafter had been fully screened and tested in accordance with the highest standards and advanced technology available and employed at that time. Armour had addressed the risk of HIV in all aspects of its process. In particular, Plasma Alliance collected plasma in low-risk centres and was at the forefront of advances in testing procedures. There is no evidence of any conduct on the part of either Dr. Rodell or Armour that would constitute wanton or reckless behaviour or a marked or substantial departure from that which is reasonable.

Heat treatment of insufficient duration and temperature

[280] It was almost universally accepted that HIV was extremely heat labile and that heat treatments of substantially shorter duration than 30 hours at 60°C would effectively inactivate any anticipated viral load. As set out above, in August and September 1986 the state of knowledge with respect to heat treatment had been established by Drs Evatt, McDougal and Petricciani. The UK withdrawal had not taken place. The exchange of screened for unscreened had taken place. Armour and Dr. Rodell were acting reasonably.

Distribution of HIV

[281] The distribution of Armour 60/30 HT Factorate continued unabated in all marketplaces globally with the exception of the United Kingdom after October 6, 1986. The designation of lots B71308, B71408 and B71508 derived from Pool #713 for Canadian export was based solely on the fact that samples of the specific lots to be exported to Canada were required to be submitted and approved by the BoB prior to its release for Canadian distribution. Lots of precisely the same product, manufactured from plasma from the same source and in accordance with precisely the same screening, look back, pooling and heat inactivation processes, were distributed throughout the world. Substantial quantities were distributed to the New York Blood Center, the largest distributor of blood products in the United States of America and the centre which employed Dr. Alfred Prince as its Head of Virology. There is no evidence of wanton or reckless conduct or of a marked or substantial departure from reasonable conduct in connection with the distribution of these lots.

Page: 60

Failed to withdraw

[282]   Every seroconversion alleged to have been associated with Armour and all meaningful inactivation studies were matters of public record. No other regulatory agency other than the DHSS recommended the withdrawal of Armour's 60/30 product. Armour was not unreasonable in failing to withdraw it.

Labelling

[283]   My finding with respect to Dr. Furesz applies here.

Failure to Notify

[284]   The continuing dialogue with worldwide regulators, the responsible investigations related to alleged seroconversion and the responsive attitude of Armour and its legion of highly qualified healthcare professionals led Armour to the rational conclusion that it was in full compliance with any required notifications relating to its product. The findings with respect to Dr. Prince apply here.

[285]   The conduct of Armour and Dr. Rodell was responsible, responsive and professional at all times. There is no element of blameworthiness that would tend to establish requisite element of wanton or reckless disregard for the lives and safety of others. It was alleged that Dr. Rodell was the directing mind of Armour. I do not make that finding for it was very clear from the evidence that decisions were made on the basis of a consensus. Interestingly, I found the conduct of all of the employees of Armour impressive. To a person, they demonstrated knowledge of the issues and care and concern for the public. I am convinced that they took the matter of public health seriously, acted responsibly and professionally. This speaks well of Armour as a corporation.

Count 5 – Common Nuisance

[286]   Armour and Dr. Rodell, are charged with the commission of a common nuisance by the distribution or failure to prevent the distribution or infusion of Armour HT Factorate thereby placing the public at risk of HIV infection.

[287]   The timeframe of the common nuisance as particularized is between April 12, 1985, the date on which Armour HT Factorate was licensed in Canada by the BoB and December 17, 1986 (it would appear that the date should read December 19, 1986, the date on which the Canadian Red Cross received the third and final lot implicated in the Canadian seroconversions). The particulars alleged mirror precisely the same allegations contained in the particulars set out in relation to counts 1 to 4 relating to the use of infected plasma, inadequate screening, look back, pooling and heat inactivation policies, the provision of an inaccurate product insert, the deficiencies in recall or withdrawal procedures and the failure to notify regulators and the public of the risk posed by HT Factorate.

Page: 61

[288]   Armour and Dr. Rodell's conduct was professional, thoughtful and responsible throughout. There is no evidence of a marked departure from that which would be reasonable in the circumstances.

[289]   The conduct of Armour and Dr. Rodell did not represent even a modest departure from conduct which was reasonable, and indeed responsible, in the circumstances. The protocol adopted by Armour in its exchange program of screened for unscreened product was endorsed by the FDA and was widely commended by the haemophiliac community.

Count 6

[290]   Armour alone is charged with failing to immediately notify the Minister of a deficiency or an alleged deficiency in its viral inactivation process as described in the studies of Dr. Alfred Prince concerning the safety of Armour HT Factorate.

[291]   The Prince experiments were so fraught with difficulties that they could not reasonably be construed to allege deficiencies in the viral inactivation process. Dr. Prince did not communicate deficiencies to Armour. As outlined above his studies produced no meaningful results. Dr. Prince did nothing to ensure that New York Blood Centre stopped distributing the HT Factorate. Neither Dr. Prince nor his studies communicated to Armour an "alleged deficiency".

[292]   Armour and Dr. Rodell are acquitted of all the charges against them.

Dr. Michael Rodell

[293]   It was alleged by the Crown that Dr. Rodell was the operating mind of Armour. He was also charged personally. Although he and Armour have been acquitted of all charges against them, a separate comment about Dr. Rodell is necessary.

[294]   As with the other defendants, Dr. Rodell has had his integrity and professionalism called into question and repeatedly attacked. I have found absolutely no conduct on his part that would warrant those attacks. The evidence established, and I believe, that Dr. Rodell has a well-deserved and eminent reputation in the medical and scientific community for his knowledge, honesty, integrity and professionalism. His colleagues admired him and to a person described him in glowing terms. The evidence confirms those assessments.

Conclusion

[295]   The evidence was detailed and extensive. It included the search for the causative agent of AIDS, the development of scientific knowledge about the virus and how to inactivate it, the treatment of haemophilia, the manufacture, licensing and distribution of blood products and the series of events up to and beyond the seroconversions in haemophiliacs. Many experts were called including highly respected scientists and physicians. People in levels of authority from administrative to high-level decision-making gave evidence.

Page: 62

[296]   Usually the passage of time is an impediment to the search for the truth. However, what was remarkable here was not what was forgotten, but what was remembered. It starts with the pain of the victims. The haemophiliacs, their families and the close-knit haemophiliac community were devastated by their losses.

[297]   The world-renowned expert on AIDS, Dr. Julio Montaner described the progression of the disease before 1996. That is when the dramatic change occurred for those infected and antiretroviral therapy became available. Before then, only the symptoms could be treated. They could be traumatic and included disfiguring lesions, warts, and oral thrush. As the opportunistic infections recurred on already damaged organs, it would lead to wasting and ultimately death. The hemophiliacs who contracted AIDS were victims. They were victims of a terrible confluence of events that they had no part in creating.

[298]   Also remembered with clarity was the struggle of the scientific and medical world, and the concern on the part of those who had to make decisions.

[299]   A conviction for criminal negligence requires conduct on the part of the accused that demonstrates wanton and reckless disregard for the lives or safety of others. A conviction for common nuisance requires conduct that represents a marked departure from that of a reasonable person in the circumstances. The circumstances at the time were established in order to judge the conduct of the accused. Their actions and their omissions were considered.

[300]   Dr. Perrault, responsible for the distribution of blood products in Canada is an expert in transfusion medicine. His conduct was cautious and careful. He consulted extensively with his highly qualified staff. During extremely difficult times, it is clear that he agonized over decisions that had to be made. Those decisions were well thought out, well supported and reasonable. Dr. Perrault was acquitted of all charges.

[301]   Dr. Furesz, responsible for the regulation of blood products in Canada is an expert in fractionation. He is highly respected both personally and professionally. In pressured situations, he made careful, reasoned and informed analysis and then did what his job required him to do: make a decision. Dr. Furesz was acquitted of all charges.

[302]   Likewise, Dr. Boucher who reported to Dr. Furesz acted reasonably throughout. Dr. Boucher was acquitted of all charges.

[303]   Armour Pharmaceutical Company, the manufacturer of the product, through its representatives, followed the scientific developments, maintained open communication with the authorities and responded quickly and responsibly when problems arose. It is clear that its corporate culture encouraged open debate, discussion and consensus-based decisions. Armour was acquitted of all charges.

[304]   Dr. Rodell, an officer of Armour was responsible and professional throughout, consistent with his well-deserved reputation for integrity. Dr. Rodell was acquitted of all charges.

Page: 63

[305]   The burden of proof in a criminal case is proof beyond a reasonable doubt. To acquit the accused on this basis however would be to "damn with faint praise".[70] There was no conduct that showed wanton and reckless disregard. There was no marked departure from the standard of a reasonable person. On the contrary, the conduct examined in detail for over one and a half years confirms reasonable, responsible and professional actions and responses during a difficult time. The allegations of criminal conduct on the part of these men and this corporation were not only unsupported by the evidence, they were disproved.

[306]   I return to the quotation of Churchill. He was speaking of events which, despite sincere efforts, turn tragic so that:

> we are so often mocked by the failure of our hopes and the upsetting of our calculations.

[307]   The events here were tragic. However, to assign blame where none exists is to compound the tragedy.

M.L. Benotto
MADAM JUSTICE M.L. BENOTTO

Released: October 1, 2007

---

[70] Borrowed from Alexander Pope: Epistle to Dr. Arbuthnot

Page: 64

Glossary Of Terms And Acronyms

60/30	Heat treatment nomenclature: heated at 60°C for 30 hours
68/72	Heat treatment nomenclature: heated at 68°C for 72 hours
AHF	Anti hemophilic factor
AIDS	Acquired immune deficiency syndrome
Assay	A test method used to measure how much HIV is present
Blood coagulation product	Product used to aid blood clotting
Blood Products Division	A division of Health Canada
BoB	Bureau of Biologics. A division of Health Canada
BTS	Blood Transfusion Service. A division of Canadian Red Cross (CRC)
CDC	Center for Disease Control (U.S.)
CRC	Canadian Red Cross
CRC-BTS	Canadian Red Cross Society's Blood Transfusion Service
DHSS	Department of Health and Social Services (U.K.)
FDA	Food and Drug Administration (U.S.)
Food and Drug Act	Canadian legislation
Fractionation	Process for separating constituent parts of blood plasma to create clotting factors
Generation I	Intermediate purity H.T. Factorate. Distributed in Canada.
Generation II	High purity H.T. Factorate. Not distributed in Canada.
H.T. Factorate	Commercial blood coagulation product manufactured by Armour
Haemophilia	Genetic disease wherein certain clotting factors as absent from the blood
Haemophilia Society	(Canada)
Heat labile	Subject to change with the addition of heat
HIV	Human Immunodeficiency Virus. The virus that causes AIDS, previously known as HTLV-III, HRI and LAV
HRI	Term previously used for HIV
HTLV-III	Term previously used for HIV
JCI	*Journal of Clinical Investigation*
Kaposi's sarcoma	Form of cancer that is generally relatively benign but was fatal to many AIDS patients in the 1980s
Krever Inquiry	Royal Commission of Inquiry on the Blood System in Canada
LAV	Term previously used for HIV
LCDC	Laboratory Centre for Disease Control. (Canadian agency in Ottawa)
Log	A measurement on a logarithmic scale
Lyophilizing	Freezing
MASAC	Medical and Scientific Advisory Council of the National Haemophilia Foundation
MMWR	Morbidity and Mortality Weekly Report. (Center for Disease Control publication)

Page: 65

National Institute for Biological Standards and Control	(U.K.)
National Institute of Health	(U.S.)
NHF	National Haemophilia Foundation (U.S.)
Phylogenetic testing	Genetic comparisons of different samples to determine whether the samples are related
Plasma	Fluid component of blood
Plasma pool	Collected plasma donations from numerous individual donors
Plasmapheresis	Removal of plasma from donors and subsequent return of red blood cells and other blood components to the donor
Product insert	Information about a pharmaceutical product provided by the manufacturer and included with the product
Viral kill	Rates used to measure viral inactivation
Viral load	Measurement of the amount of a particular virus in the blood (or other bodily fluid) of a given individual
Viral titre	Concentration of virus in a particular sample

| Requiem For Critical Thinking?

The multiplication of case studies, like the one developed in this volume, is meant to both put some order in complex files, and to suggest ways to design more effective methods to deal with such matters. And it is also intended to smoke out the broader debilitating forces at work that might undermine our social learning abilities in general, and enfeeble our capability to deal effectively with any problem with which we might be confronted.

Our analysis of the tainted-blood tragedy has revealed the existence of such sources of social learning disabilities. The most important one is probably the demise of critical thinking – something we have noticed at all levels in the tainted-blood affair but also in many other contexts and files (Paquet 2014). This sort of *molle pensée* has been responsible for the failure to develop a meaningful appreciative system, capable of grappling with the growing complexity of modern organizations and institutions.

This weakness has undermined the whole process of description of the setting and circumstances of the issues of interest, thwarted the process of problem definition, and derailed the development of the multidimensional frameworks required to take into account the divergence of viewpoints. Ultimately, it has weakened efforts to nudge into existence the requisite blending of perspectives, capable of generating the appropriate trade-offs among the views of crucial partners to ensure commitment to collaborative governance and effective wayfinding.

Moreover, it has enfeebled the whole process of inquiring and social learning in good currency – i.e., the process of knowledge production necessary to fuel the continuous adjustment of organizations to the contextual change, and to the evolving changes in the needs and preferences of the different stakeholders. Thus, it has prevented the emergence of the new modes of production of knowledge required to ensure the progress and survivability of organizations through the learning of new means, new ends, and the experimentation with new organizational designs calling for a modification of their very fabric and mission.

Failure of critical thinking has undermined mindfulness and social learning. Initiatives have been proposed to correct the situation, but they have emerged with great slowness and clumsiness. Consequently, the resilience and survivability of the organizations have been threatened.

Critical thinking is a *manière de voir*, a commitment not to put up with bullshit as Frankfurt (2005) would have put it, an engagement to ask always and systematically why and how, and a commitment to insist on maintaining a mindfulness that is persistently and relentlessly vigilant – continually and in all circumstances. This vigilance is the only way to enhance the integrity of the process of inquiry itself that requires thinking skills, a skeptic's worldview, and a commitment to intellectual due process in a manner that is as free of failure and slippage as possible. However, this is too general a way of stating what has to be done.

A more specific way to proceed is to recognize that the flaws at the source of poor critical thinking might be regarded as resulting in three major blockages: poor critical description of the context and the organization, mental prisons preventing as extensive an examination of the issues as possible, and poor appreciation of the socio-ethical constraints in good currency in a particular social system.

One cannot presume that a taste for critical thinking can be regenerated overnight after a long period when it has been systematically discouraged, and has gone into hibernation. It would be equally naïve to believe that a design attitude will emerge instantaneously.

Ground zero is a mindfulness that fosters critical thinking and learning.

Phase I is a greater awareness of the cost of the erosion of critical thinking that leads to a sanitization of language, a refusal to confront head on even the worst sophistry and deception, and an acceptance of even the most unreasonable accommodation in the name of tolerance. This awareness would ensure a vibrant capability to detect collaborative breakdowns, and any form of derailment of the social order ascribable to disinformation or information cascades.

Phase II is the recognition both that there are reasons to be concerned about these developments, and that their causes and sources need to be probed. This, in turn, calls for the highest and best use of irony and irreverence to challenge the assemblage of disingenuity and sophistry that is currently posturing as conventional wisdom in academe and elsewhere. Nothing less than methodological and intellectual cruelty is required. How else can one hope to awaken those who only pretend to sleep?

Phase III is the behavioural change that will reinstate the former natural proclivity of citizens to ask why and how as a matter of course. A gentle first step might be a campaign to encourage the questioning of all assumptions. But this will not suffice. What must be mustered is the courage and audacity to declare an open season for the slaughtering of sacred cows: humanely, but relentlessly and mercilessly ... one at a time ... every day ... (Paquet 2014: chaper 1).

How does one accomplish this?

The most important way is through the preservation of loci where critical thinking is encouraged, and a virulent reaction to the weakening of any such loci – such as the fact that a publicly funded university press rejected a very detailed and informative study by a respected academic questioning the unbounded alarmism about climate change (Hart 2015). Such capitulation to the tyranny of conventional wisdom and the hegemony of *pouvoir social à la* Tocqueville – a dominant public opinion however ill-founded becoming a reference that paralyzes criticism and intimidates stakeholders to the point of becoming a form of discreet censorship (Boudon 2005: 168) – is unacceptable.[10]

Modern societies will be faced with more and more crises in the future akin to the tainted-blood tragedy, and unless we learn all the lessons from that tragedy (including the lack of critical thinking throughout) and act boldly upon those lessons learned, we are bound to repeat the awful mistakes echoed above.

Not to act with gumption now – by at the very least a major investment in developing our critical thinking – could only be regarded as "an unsettling or rash lack of concern" or (more brutally in the other official language) *"une insouciance déréglée ou téméraire"* – the definition of criminal negligence in the Canadian Criminal Code!

---

[10] The Centre on Governance of the University of Ottawa has been such a locus for critical thinking about ways to govern for the last 20 years, a locus of choice for questioning all assumptions and for proposing heretical responses to governance problems. The COG has (1) developed new approaches to governance, (2) encouraged critical thinking, irreverence, and experimentation as the most promising road to systematically exposing pathologies of governance in all its forms in private, public and social organizations, and (3) provided effective repairs for them. At a time when rekindling critical thinking would appear to be the order of the day, one might benefit from taking a look at the more than 70 books and reports the COG has produced with this sole purpose in mind since 1997. A list is available at the end of this volume.

References

Boudon, Raymond. 2005. *Tocqueville aujourd'hui*. Paris, FR: Odile Jacob.

Frankfurt, Harry G. 2005. *On Bullshit*. Princeton, NJ: Princeton University Press.

Hart, Michael. 2015. *Hubris – The troubling science, economics, and politics of climate change*. Ottawa, ON: Compleat Desktops Publishing.

Paquet, Gilles. 2014. *Unusual Suspects – Essays on Social Learning Disabilities*. Ottawa, ON: Invenire.

ADDENDUM

| About the Centre on Governance of the University of Ottawa

The Centre on Governance (COG) was created by Gilles Paquet at the end of 1997 as a joint venture of the Faculty of Administration (now the Telfer School of Management) and the Faculty of Social Sciences at the University of Ottawa. From its inception, it was seen as an umbrella organization – a hub for the work on governance taking place in all the faculties of the University of Ottawa. The main objectives of the Centre were to develop: conceptual frameworks for analyzing coordination problems, tools to better analyze governance issues, and a critical approach for repairing governance failures. It was meant to bring together persons who are committed to seeking better responses to contemporary problems of governance in the private, public and civic sectors both within and outside of the University of Ottawa. It aimed from the beginning to be an observatory of emerging trends and experiments in the world of governance.

From the beginning, the COG has been responsible for the publication of *www.optimumonline.ca* – a refereed quarterly on governance and public management. Fellows of the Centre have produced hundreds of papers over the years and generated large numbers of books published under different banners. What follows is a list of the main books and reports produced by the Centre, under the banner of the University of Ottawa Press, then under the banner of Invenire – The Idea Factory, and also under the banners of other publishers. All these books are available from www.amazon.ca.

The University of Ottawa Press (1999-2010)

D. McInnes. 1999. *Taking it to the Hill – The Complete Guide to Appearing before Parliamentary Committees*

G. Paquet. 1999. *Governance through Social Learning*

L. Cardinal & C. Andrew (sld). 2001. *La démocratie à l'épreuve de la gouvernance*

L. Cardinal & D. Headon (eds.). 2002. *Shaping Nations – Constitutionalism and Society in Australia and Canada*

P. Boyer *et al.* (eds.). 2004. *From Subjects to Citizens – A hundred years of citizenship in Australia and Canada*

C. Andrew *et al.* (eds.). 2005. *Accounting for Culture – Thinking though Cultural Citizenship*

G. Paquet. 2005. *The New Geo-Governance: A Baroque Approach*

J. Roy. 2005. *E-government in Canada*

C. Rouillard *et al.* 2006. *Re-engineering the State – Toward an Impoverishment of Quebec Governance*

E. Brunet-Jailly (ed.). 2007. *Borderlands – Comparing Border Security in North America and Europe*

R, Hubbard & G. Paquet. 2007. *Gomery's Blinders and Canadian Federalism*

N. Brown & L. Cardinal (eds.). 2007. *Managing Diversity – Practices of Citizenship*

J. Roy. 2007. *Business and Government in Canada*

T. Brzustowski. 2008. *The Way Ahead – Meeting Canada's Productivity Challenge*

G. Paquet. 2008. *Tableau d'avancement – Petite ethnographie interprétative d'un certain Canada français*

P. Schafer. 2008. *Revolution or Renaissance – Making the transition from an economic age to a cultural age*

G. Paquet. 2008. *Deep Cultural Diversity – A Governance Challenge*

L. Juillet & K. Rasmussen. 2008. *A la défense d'un idéal contesté – le principe de mérite et la CFP 1908-2008*

L. Juillet & K. Rasmussen. 2008. *Defending a Contested Ideal – Merit and the Public Service Commission 1908-2008*

C. Andrew *et al.* (eds.). *Gilles Paquet – Homo Hereticus*

O.P. Dvivedi *et al.* (eds.). 2009. *The Evolving Physiology of Government – Canadian Public Administration in Transition*

G. Paquet. 2009. *Crippling Epistemologies and Governane Failures – A Plea for Experimentalism*

M. Small. 2009. *The Forgotten Peace – Mediation at Niagara Falls 1914*

R. Hubbard & G. Paquet. 2010. *The Black Hole of Public Administration*

P. Dutil *et al.* 2010. *The Service State: Rhetoric, Reality, and Promises*

G. DiGiacomo & M. Flumian (eds.). 2010. *The Case for Centralized Federalism*

R. Hubbard & G. Paquet (eds.). 2010. *The Case for Decentralized Federalism*

Invenire (2009-2016)

R. Higham. 2009. *Who do we think we are: Canada's reasonable (and less reasonable) accommodation debates*

R. Hubbard. 2009. *Profession: Public Servant*

G. Paquet. 2009. *Scheming Virtuously: The Road to Collaborative Governance*

J. Bowen (ed.). 2009. *The Entrepreneurial Effect: Ottawa*

F. Lapointe. 2011. *Cities as Crucibles: Reflections on Canada's Urban Future*

J. Bowen. 2011. *The Entrepreneurial Effect: Waterloo*

G. Paquet. 2011. *Tableau d'avancement II – Essais exploratoires sur la gouvernance d'un certain Canada français*

R. Chattopadhyay & G. Paquet (eds.). 2011. *The Unimagined Canadian Capital – Challenges for the Federal Capital Region*

P. Camu. 2011. *La Flotte Blanche – Histoire de la Compagnie de la navigation du Richelieu et d'Ontario 1845-1913*

M. Behiels & F. Rocher (eds.). 2011. *The State in Transition – Challenges for Canadian Federalism*

R. Clément & C. Andrew (eds.). 2012. *Cities and Languages: Governance and Policy – International Symposium*

R. Clément & C. Andrew (sld). 2012. *Villes et langues : gouvernance et politiques – Symposium international*

C.M. Rocan. 2012. *Challenges in Public Health Governance: The Canadian Experience*

T. Brzustowski. 2012. *Why we need more innovation in Canada and what we must do to get it*

C. Andrew *et al.* 2012. *Gouvernance comunautaire : innovations dans le Canada français hors Québec*

M. Gervais. 2012. *Challenges of Minority Governments in Canada*

R. Hubbard *et al.* (eds.). 2012. *Stewardship: Collaborative decentred metagovernance and inquiring systems*

G. Paquet. 2012. *Moderato cantabile: Toward principled governance for Canada's immigration policy*

G. Paquet & T. Ragan. 2012. *Through the Detox Prism: Exploring organizational failures and design responses*

G. Paquet. 2013. *Tackling Wicked Policy Problems: Equality, Diversity, and Sustainability*

G. Paquet. 2013. *Gouvernance corporative : une entrée en matières*

G. Paquet. 2014. *Tableau d'avancement III – Pour une diaspora canadienne-française antifragile*

R. Clément & P. Foucher. 2014. *50 years of official bilingualism: challenges, analyses and testimonies*

R. Clément & P. Foucher. 2014. *50 ans de bilinguisme official : défis, analyses et témoignages*

R. Hubbard & G. Paquet. 2014. *Probing the Bureaucratic Mind: About Canadian Federal Executives*

G. Paquet. 2014. *Unusual Suspects: Essays on Social Learning Disabilities*

R. Hubbard & G. Paquet. 2015. *Irregular Governance: A Plea for Bold Organizational Experimentation*

L. Cardinal & P. Devette (eds.). 2015. *Autour de Chantal Mouffe – Le politique en conflit*

R. Higham. 2015. *What would you say? ... as guest speaker at the next Canadian citizenship ceremony*

D. Gordon. 2015. *Town and Crown – An Illustrated History of Canada's Capital*

G. Paquet & R.A. Perrault. 2016. *The Tainted-Blood Tragedy in Canada: A Cascade of Governance Failures*

G. Paquet & C. Wilson. 2016. *Intelligent Governance: A Prototype for Social Coordination*

Editions Liber

G. Paquet. 1999. *Oublier la Révolution tranquille – Pour une nouvelle socialité*

G. Paquet. 2004. *Pathologies de gouvernance – Essais de technologie sociale*

G. Paquet. 2005. *Gouvernance : une invitation à la subversion*

G. Paquet. 2008. *Gouvernance : mode d'emploi*

G. Paquet. 2011. *Gouvernance collaborative : un anti-manuel*

Éditions Vrin

P. Laurent & G. Paquet. 1998. *Épistémologie et économie de la relation – coordination et gouvernance distribuée*

Éditions H.M.H.

G. Paquet & J.P. Wallot. 2007. *Un Québec moderne 1760-1840 : Essai d'histoire économique et sociale*

Government of Canada

G. Paquet. 2006 (en collaboration). *The National Capital Commission: Charting a New Course*

Report of the NCC Mandate Review Panel

Special research reports

COG, 1999. *The Borough Model: Municipal Restructuring for Ottawa*

COG, 2000. *The Governance of the Ethical Process for Research – A study for the Tri-council*

COG, 2000. *Governance in the 21st Century* (The Royal Society of Canada)

G. Paquet. 2001. *Si Montfort m'était conté...Essais de pathologie administrative et de rétroprospective*

A. Chaiton & G. Paquet (eds.). 2002. *Ottawa 2020 – A synthesis of the Smart Growth Summit*

G. Paquet & Kevin Wilkins. 2002. *Ocean governance... An inquiry into stakeholding*